# Low Fodmap Diet Cookbook

# Table of Contents

# 50 Vegetarian Recipes

## Low FODMAP Yellow Snack Cake with Rainbow Sprinkles

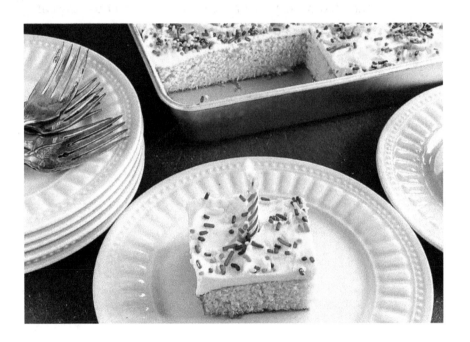

Makes: 24 Servings Prep Time: 10 minutes Total Time: 10 minutes

INGREDIENTS:

1 recipe Yellow Cake, baked in a 13-inch by 9-inch (33 cm by 23 cm) pan and cooled

1 batch Swiss Meringue Buttercream, freshly made and ready to use

Sprinkles; optional

Birthday candles; optional

PREPARATION:

Take out the cake from the pan. Frost your cake with buttercream. Sprinkle different sprinkles over your cake. Let it set and your cake is ready to serve.

If you are traveling somewhere with your cake then you do not need to take out a cake from the pan. Just decorate it in the pan and take it with you.

NUTRITION

Calories: 391kcal | Carbohydrates: 42g | Protein: 3g | Fat: 24g

# Low FODMAP Coconut Lime Bread

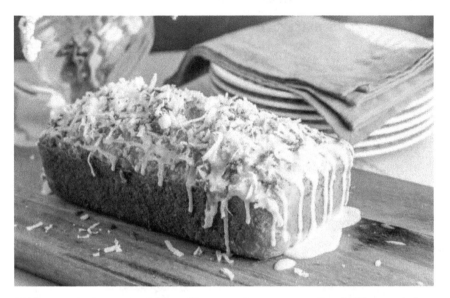

Makes: 12 Servings Prep Time: 10 minutes Cook Time: 1 hour

Total Time: 1 hour 10 minutes

INGREDIENTS:

Bread:

1 1/3 cups (194 g) low FODMAP gluten-free all-purpose flour, such as Bob's Red Mill 1 to 1 Gluten-Free Baking Flour

1 cup (198 g) sugar

1 teaspoon baking powder; use gluten-free if following a gluten-free diet

½ teaspoon salt

¾ cup (180 ml) canned full-fat coconut milk, at room temperature

½ cup (120 ml) unrefined coconut oil, melted and cooled

2 large eggs

2 tablespoons very fine lime zest, made with a rasp-style zester

1 tablespoon freshly squeezed lime juice

1 teaspoon vanilla extract

½ cup (38 g) plus 2 tablespoons sweetened flaked coconut, divided

Glaze & Topping:

1 cup (90 g) sifted confectioner's sugar

2 tablespoons freshly squeezed lime juice

2 tablespoons sweetened flaked coconut

1 tablespoon very fine lime zest, made with a rasp-style zester

PREPARATION:

For the bread:

Pre-heat your oven at 350°F (180°C). Line 8 ½-inch by 4 ¼-inch pan with parchment paper. Overhang the two sides and coat the paper and set aside.

Mix the flour, sugar, baking powder, and salt. Make a well in the center. In a separate bowl place the coconut milk, coconut oil, eggs, lime zest and juice, and vanilla extract and whisk together well.

Mix wet ingredients to dry ingredients and fold well. After it's done put the mixture in a pan. Place the loaf pan in the oven to bake the bread. Bake for at least 30 minutes. When it's done take it out and decorate with topping.

For topping:

Mix sugar and lime juice well together. Drizzle this glaze over cool bread. Let it set and then sprinkle lemon zest over it. The bread is ready to serve.

NUTRITION

Calories: 328kcal | Carbohydrates: 48g | Protein: 2g | Fat: 15g | Saturated Fat: 3g | Cholesterol: 3mg | Sodium: 172mg | Potassium: 44mg | Fiber: 2g | Sugar: 32g | Calcium: 1mg | Iron: 1mm

# Low FODMAP Smoked Gouda Apple Muffins

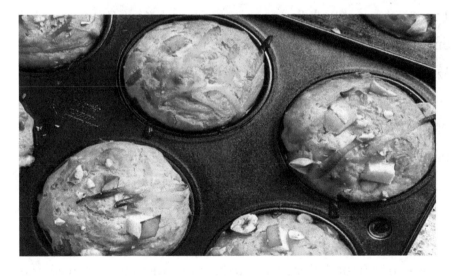

Makes: 12 Servings Prep Time: 10 minutes Cook Time: 15 minutes Total Time: 25 minutes

INGREDIENTS:

1 cup (240 ml) lactose-free whole milk, at room temperature

1 tablespoon lemon juice

2 cups (290 g) low FODMAP gluten-free all-purpose flour, such as Bob's Red Mill 1 to 1 Gluten-Free Baking Flour

1 ½ teaspoon baking powder; use gluten-free if following a gluten-free diet

½ teaspoon baking soda

¼ teaspoon salt

3 large eggs, at room temperature

½ cup (107 g) firmly packed light brown sugar

1/3 cup (75 ml) extra-virgin olive oil

1 medium-sized Pink Lady apple cored and diced (leave the peel on)

½ cup (50 g) chopped toasted, skinned hazelnuts

5- ounces (140 g) smoked gouda, shredded

PREPARATION:

Position rack in center of oven. Preheat oven to 425°F (220°C). Line 12 muffin cups with paper liners or coat with nonstick spray. Mix lemon juice and milk well and set them aside to thicken. It takes around 5 minutes.

Besides mix flour, baking soda, baking powder, and salt in a large bowl. Make a well in a center and place it aside.

Beat brown sugar and eggs along with prepared sour milk and olive oil. Beat this mixture until it gets smooth.

Combine the dry ingredients with the wet mixture. Fold it well and add nuts, apple, and cheese. Put this mixture in a muffins tray to bake.

Bake muffins for 12 to 15 minutes or until you press a toothpick and it comes out clean. After getting done take them out and serve.

NUTRITION

Calories: 301kcal | Carbohydrates: 33g | Protein: 7g | Fat: 16g | Saturated Fat: 1g | Sodium: 226mg | Potassium: 16mg | Fiber: 1g | Sugar: 11g | Vitamin A: 8IU | Vitamin C: 1mg | Calcium: 1mg | Iron: 1mg

# Low FODMAP Beer Bread

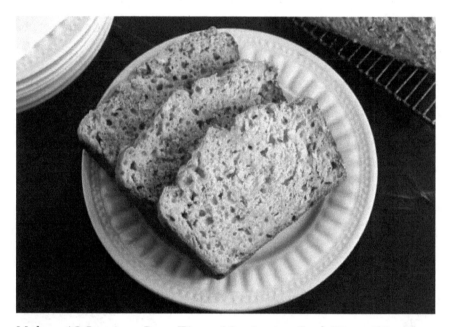

Makes: 12 Servings Prep Time: 10 minutes Cook Time: 50 minutes

Total Time: 1 hour

INGREDIENTS:

2 ½ cups (363 g) low FODMAP gluten-free all-purpose flour, such as Bob's Red Mill 1 to 1 Gluten-Free Baking Flour

½ cup (50 g) old-fashioned rolled oats; use gluten-free if following a gluten-free diet

1 tablespoon baking powder; use gluten-free if following a gluten-free diet

1 tablespoon sugar

1 teaspoon caraway seeds; optional

1 teaspoon salt

3 large eggs, at room temperature

3 tablespoons honey

3 tablespoons extra-virgin olive oil

12- ounce (360 ml) bottle or can of beer; use gluten-free if following a gluten-free diet

¼ cup (16 g) chopped scallions, green parts only; optional

½ cup (55 g) shredded cheddar cheese; divided and optional (I like sharp orange-colored cheddar)

PREPARATION:

Position rack in the middle of the oven. Preheat oven to 375°F (190°C). Coat a 9-inch by 5-inch (23 cm by 12 cm) loaf pan with nonstick spray, line the bottom with parchment paper allowing it to overhand the two short ends, then coat paper.

Whisk flour, baking powder, oats, sugar, and salt well in a big mixing bowl.

In other bowl mix eggs, honey and oil. Whisk this mixture well and add it to dry ingredients. Fold all mixture well until a smooth mixture is formed. After this add beer and fold again the mixture. Put the pan in the oven and bake it for 20 minutes. Take out and sprinkle cheese and again bake for 20 minutes or until the top gets golden brown. Take out the pan and let it cool. Take out the bread from the pan and serve.

NUTRITION

Calories: 267kcal | Carbohydrates: 40g | Protein: 6g | Fat: 7g | Saturated Fat: 1g | Sodium: 327mg | Potassium: 36mg | Fiber: 2g | Sugar: 5g | Calcium: 6mg | Iron: 1mg

## Low FODMAP Hazelnut Shortcake with Berries & Caramel

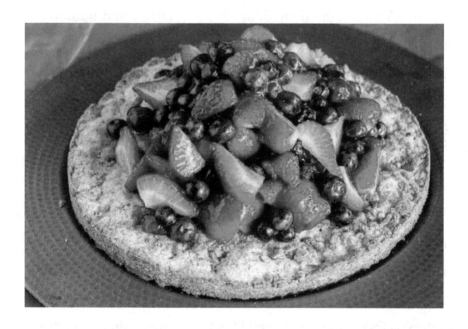

Makes: 8 Servings Prep Time: 20 minutes Cook Time: 30 minutes Total Time: 50 minutes

INGREDIENTS:

Hazelnut Shortcake:

2- ounces (55 g) skinned, toasted hazelnuts

1 2/3 cups (241 g) low FODMAP gluten-free all-purpose flour, such as Bob's Red Mill 1 to 1 Baking Flour

¼ cup (54 g) plus 1 tablespoon firmly packed light brown sugar, divided

1 tablespoon baking powder; use gluten-free if following a gluten-free diet

½ teaspoon salt

1 cup (240 ml) lactose-free heavy cream

Berry Topping:

10- ounces (280 g) fresh strawberries, hulled and halved or quartered (depending on size), at room temperature

6- ounces (170 g) fresh blueberries, at room temperature

3- ounces (85 g) fresh raspberries, at room temperature

2- ounces (55 g) fresh blackberries, at room temperature

½ cup (120 ml) Low FODMAP Salted Caramel Sauce, fluid and ready to use

PREPARATION:

For the Shortcake: Position rack in the middle of the oven. Preheat oven to 400°F (200°C). Coat the inside of a 9-inch (23 cm) round springform pan with nonstick spray; set aside.

Grind nuts in the food processor by turning the button on and off. Put it in a bowl and add flour, baking powder, brown sugar, and salt. Mix all these ingredients well. Pour cream and mix well until a soft dough is formed.

Place this dough on a baking tray with fingers. Add remaining brown sugar on the top and bake it for 30 minutes. When it's done take it out and place it on the rack and cool down.

For the Filling & Assembly: Place all of the berries in a mixing bowl. Pour caramel sauce over the berries and fold gently, then mound on top of the shortcake. Serve immediately, cut into wedges.

NUTRITION

Calories: 386kcal | Carbohydrates: 54g | Protein: 4g | Fat: 14g | Sodium: 277mg | Fiber: 2g | Sugar: 9g

# Low FODMAP Fluffy Pancakes

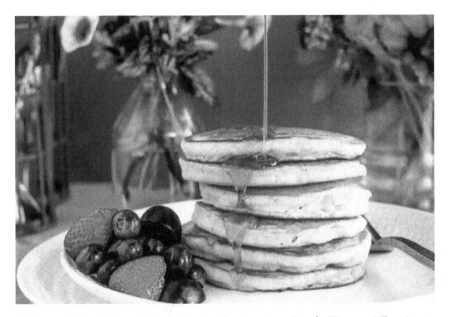

Makes: 8 Servings Prep Time: 5 minutes Cook Time: 15 minutes Total Time: 20 minutes

INGREDIENTS:

2 cups (290 g) low FODMAP, gluten-free all-purpose flour, such as Bob's Red Mill 1 to 1 Gluten-Free Baking Flour

¼ cup (50 g) sugar

1 tablespoon plus 1 teaspoon baking powder; use gluten-free if following a gluten-free diet

½ teaspoon salt

¼ teaspoon baking soda

1 ¾ cups (420 ml) whole lactose-free milk, at room temperature

¼ cup (57 g; ½ stick) melted unsalted butter, cooled to just warm

1 large egg, at room temperature

1 teaspoon vanilla extract

PREPARATION:

Stir flour, baking powder, sugar, salt, and baking soda in a large bowl. Mix the wet ingredients in a separate bowl.

Mix all of the wet mixtures into dry ingredients and fold well.

Place a non-stick pan overheat. Spread the batter on the pan and cook on medium heat. Cook it until bubbles are formed and the bottom gets golden brown. Turn it and cook from another side as well. Serve it with hot maple syrup.

NUTRITION

Calories: 253kcal | Carbohydrates: 41g | Protein: 5g | Fat: 8g | Sodium: 319mg | Fiber: 1g | Sugar: 10g

# LOW FODMAP SUN-DRIED TOMATO PESTO

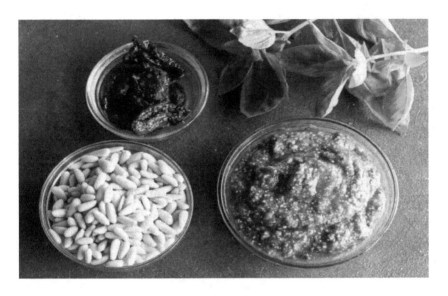

Makes: 8 Servings Prep Time: 10 minutes Total Time: 10 minutes

INGREDIENTS:

2 cups (16 g) fresh basil leaves

1 cup (100 g) grated Parmesan cheese

½ cup (76 g) lightly toasted European pine nuts, cooled

1 ¾- ounces (50 g) flexible sun-dried tomatoes

1 teaspoon kosher salt or to taste

1 cup (240 ml) Garlic-Infused Oil, made with olive oil, or purchased equivalent

PREPARATION:

Place basil, cheese, pine nuts, sun-dried tomatoes, and 1 teaspoon salt in a food processor fitted with a metal blade. Pulse on and off until finely chopped. Turn on the machine and add oil slowly and continue processing until a smooth paste is formed. Taste the mixture and add seasoning according to it. It is ready to use. You can refrigerate it for 2 weeks.

NUTRITION

Calories: 442kcal | Carbohydrates: 8g | Protein: 15g | Fat: 41g | Saturated Fat: 5g | Cholesterol: 26mg | Sodium: 455mg | Potassium: 211mg | Fiber: 2g | Sugar: 1g | Vitamin A: 3376IU | Vitamin C: 11mg | Calcium: 433mg | Iron: 2mg

# LOW FODMAP MASALA CHAI

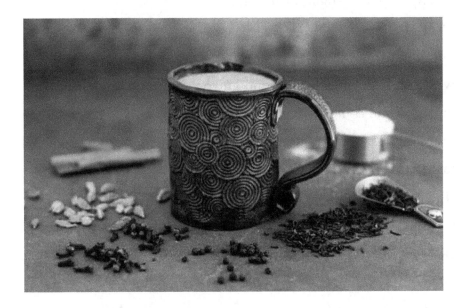

Makes: 2 Servings Prep Time: 2 minutes Cook Time: 6 minutes

Total Time: 8 minutes

INGREDIENTS:

1 ½ cups (360 ml) water

2 green cardamom pods

1 whole clove

1 whole black peppercorn

1/16 teaspoon ground cinnamon

Pinch ground ginger; optional

1/8- ounce (4 g) loose black tea, such as a hearty Assam

¼ cup to ½ cup (60 ml to 120 ml) lactose-free whole milk; or to taste

1 to 3 teaspoons sugar; or to taste

PREPARATION:

Put water in a pot and place it overheat. Add cardamoms along with peppercorn, clove, ground ginger, and cinnamon. Add your loose tea and cook for 3 minutes.

Add milk as much milky tea as you want and add some sugar to taste. Serve it immediately in cups.

NUTRITION

Calories: 42kcal | Carbohydrates: 7g | Protein: 2g | Fat: 1g | Saturated Fat: 1g | Sodium: 10mg | Potassium: 34mg | Fiber: 1g | Sugar: 4g | Vitamin C: 1mg | Calcium: 17mg | Iron: 1mg

# VEGAN LOW FODMAP CRISP TOPPING

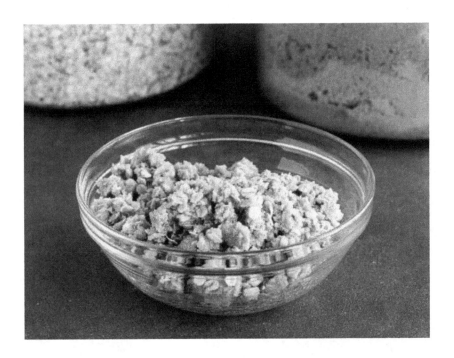

Makes: 8 Servings Prep Time: 10 minutes Total Time: 10 minutes

INGREDIENTS:

¾ cup (160 g) firmly packed light brown sugar

¾ cup (109 g) low FODMAP gluten-free flour, such as Bob's Red Mill Gluten Free 1 to 1 Baking Flour

¾ cup (74 g) old-fashioned rolled oats (not instant or quick oats); use gluten-free if following a gluten-free diet

¼ teaspoon cinnamon

¼ teaspoon salt

½ cup (120 ml) melted coconut oil, either refined or unrefined

PREPARATION:

Put sugar, oats, cinnamon, flour, and salt in a bowl and mix well. Add melted oil and stir until all mixture gets mixed. The crisp is ready to use.

NUTRITION

Calories: 268kcal | Carbohydrates: 35g | Protein: 2g | Fat: 15g | Sodium: 73mg | Fiber: 1g | Sugar: 18g

# LOW FODMAP PEACHES AND CREAM POPSICLES WITH RASPBERRIES

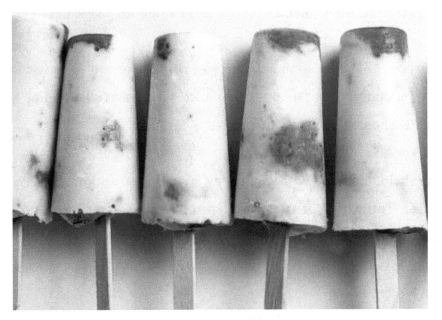

Makes: 8 Servings Prep Time: 15 minutes Freeze Time: 8 hours

Total Time: 8 hours 15 minutes

**INGREDIENTS:**

8 ½- ounces (240 g) chopped peaches, peeled stones discarded; buy 3 peaches to be safe

1 cup (245 g) thick vanilla lactose-free yogurt

1 tablespoon plus 1 teaspoon honey, divided

½ teaspoon lemon juice, divided

2 ¾- ounces (75 g) fresh raspberries

**PREPARATION:**

Chop peaches and add them to a blender along with lime juice, yogurt, and honey. Blend it well to form a smooth paste. Get ready the mold of your popsicles.

In a small bowl mash the raspberries with 1 teaspoon honey and the remaining ¼ teaspoon lemon juice. Spoon a small amount of the mashed raspberries into each pop mold.

Fill molds halfway with yogurt/peach mixture, add more berry purée. Top with more yogurt mixture. Insert wooden sticks that come with your popsicle set. Freeze it overnight and it is ready to eat.

**NUTRITION**

Calories: 49kcal | Carbohydrates: 10g | Protein: 2g | Fat: 1g | Sodium: 1mg | Fiber: 2g | Sugar: 7g | Vitamin C: 1mg

# LOW FODMAP NO-CHURN VANILLA ICE CREAM WITH CHOCOLATE COVERED ALMONDS

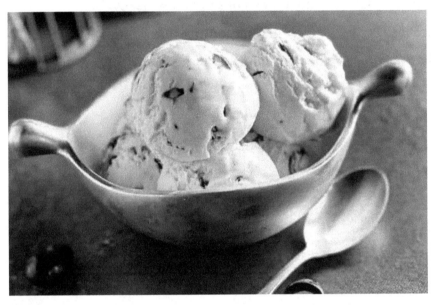

Makes: 10 Servings Prep Time: 15 minutes Dairy Resting Time & Chilling Time: 16 hours Total Time: 16 hours 15 minutes

**INGREDIENTS:**

2 cups (480 ml) lactose-free heavy cream, chilled

½ cup (99 g) sugar; use superfine if you have it

1 vanilla bean, split

1 tablespoon whiskey

Pinch salt

½ cup (90 g) dark chocolate covered almonds (about 22 nuts), chopped

**PREPARATION:**

Put chilled cream and sugar in a mixer. Add vanilla bean seeds into the mixture. Add a pinch of salt and whiskey. Beat it with an electric beater. After getting done fold it in chopped dark chocolate covered almonds. Put it in a container and freeze overnight.

**NUTRITION**

Calories: 251kcal | Carbohydrates: 17g | Protein: 1g | Fat: 12g | Sodium: 1mg | Sugar: 12g

# LOW FODMAP NO-CHURN VANILLA ICE CREAM

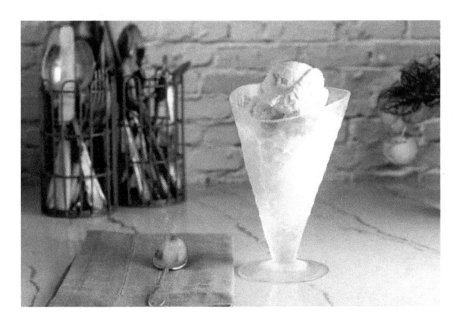

Makes: 10 Servings Prep Time: 15 minutes Dairy Resting Time & Chilling Time: 16 hours Total Time: 16 hours 15 minutes

**INGREDIENTS:**

2 cups (480 ml) lactose-free heavy cream, chilled

2 teaspoons vanilla extract

Pinch salt

1, 14- ounce (397 g) can lactose-free sweetened condensed milk

PREPARATION:

Mix chilled cream, vanilla, and salt in a large mixing bowl. Beat this mixture with an electric mixer Take care not to over-beat it.

Put it into an airtight container and freeze until firm, preferably overnight. Allow sitting for a few minutes at room temperature. Serve and enjoy immediately as it melts faster than conventional ice cream.

**NUTRITION**

Calories: 296kcal | Carbohydrates: 24g | Protein: 4g | Fat: 14g | Sodium: 1mg | Sugar: 1g

# LOW FODMAP CANTALOUPE, CUCUMBER AND BURRATA SALAD

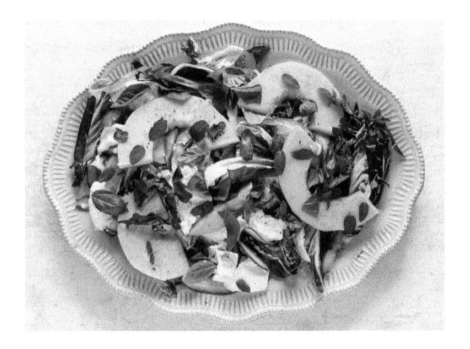

Makes: 8 Servings Prep Time: 15 minutes Total Time: 15 minutes

**INGREDIENTS:**

2- pounds (910 g) peeled, seeded, sliced ripe cantaloupe

Kosher salt

Freshly ground black pepper

1 small head (about 300 g) radicchio, cored and cut or torn into bite-sized pieces

3 Persian cucumbers, trimmed, sliced into wide, thin ribbons

8- ounces (225 g) burrata; typically about 2 pieces

Fresh basil leaves; a small handful

Fresh mint leaves; a small handful

Low FODMAP Red Wine Vinaigrette

**PREPARATION:**

Have a bowl or platter to set a salad. First of all place melon around the platter. Arrange radicchio over the melon. Now decorate the top with cucumbers.

Cut the burrata into a bite-sized piece and put it at the top so that liquid can be spilled over. Cut and tear herbs and spread over salad. You can refrigerate it and it is ready to serve.

**NUTRITION**

Calories: 129kcal | Carbohydrates: 15g | Protein: 6g | Fat: 7g | Saturated Fat: 1g | Sodium: 1mg | Potassium: 31mg | Fiber: 2g | Sugar: 13g | Vitamin A: 22IU | Vitamin C: 1mg | Calcium: 3mg | Iron: 1mg

# LOW FODMAP CARROT-GINGER SOUP

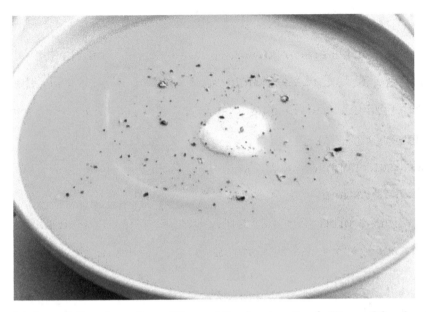

Makes: 8 Servings Prep Time: 10 minutes Cook Time: 30 minutes

Total Time: 40 minutes

**INGREDIENTS:**

1 teaspoon extra-virgin olive oil or butter

½ cup coarsely chopped fennel bulb

1 medium celery stalk, coarsely chopped

2 tablespoons grated peeled fresh ginger, plus more as needed

6 cups Nourishing Vegetable Broth, from the book or use our Low

FODMAP Vegetable Broth

6 medium carrots, peeled and coarsely chopped

2 medium yellow potatoes, coarsely chopped

¼ teaspoon freshly ground black pepper plus more as needed

¼ teaspoon salt plus more as needed (optional)

½ cup vegan yogurt, optional

**PREPARATION:**

In a large pot, heat the oil over medium-high heat. Add the fennel and celery, and sauté for 5 minutes, or until softened. Reduce the heat to medium. Add the ginger, and cook, stirring constantly, for 2 minutes.

Add carrots, pepper, potatoes, broth, and salt in a pot. Bring it to the boil. Cover and cook until potatoes get tender.

Using a food processor blend the soup mixture to form puree consistency. Taste and add seasonings according to your taste. Serve it immediately.

**NUTRITION**

Calories: 69kcal | Carbohydrates: 14g | Protein: 1g | Fat: 1g | Sodium: 73mg | Fiber: 2g | Sugar: 3g

# LOW FODMAP TOFU SALAD

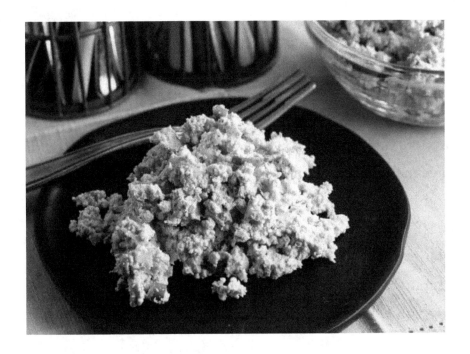

Makes: 6 Servings Prep Time: 5 minutes Freezing Time: 8 hours

Total Time: 8 hours 5 minutes

**INGREDIENTS:**

14- ounce (400 g) container of the firm or extra-firm tofu in water

½ cup (113 g) mayonnaise

2 teaspoons Dijon mustard

2 teaspoons lemon juice

1 medium carrot, peeled and shredded

1 medium stalk celery, finely diced

2 tablespoons chopped scallions, green parts only

Kosher salt

Freshly ground black pepper

Dulse flakes; optional

**PREPARATION:**

Put tofu in the freezer overnight. Take it out and crumble it. Press tofu to take out as much water as you can.

Put tofu in a mixing bowl and add mustard, lemon juice, mayonnaise, carrot, scallion greens, and celery. Mix it and taste it according to your taste. It is ready to serve.

**NUTRITION**

Calories: 206kcal | Carbohydrates: 3g | Protein: 7g | Fat: 18g | Saturated Fat: 2g | Cholesterol: 8mg | Sodium: 144mg | Fiber: 1g | Sugar: 1g | Vitamin A: 13IU | Vitamin C: 1mg | Iron: 1mg

# LOW FODMAP ORANGE CARROT JUICE

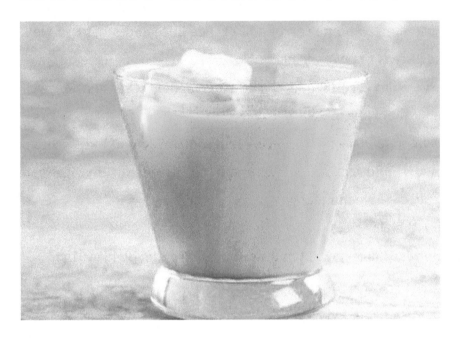

Makes: 2 Servings Prep Time: 5 minutes Total Time: 5 minutes

**INGREDIENTS:**

Basic Blend:

½ cup (120 ml) freshly squeezed carrot juice

½ cup (120 ml) freshly squeezed orange juice

Add-Ons:

¼ cup (60 ml) UHT unsweetened coconut milk

2 tablespoons low FODMAP whey protein isolate, such as Opportunities Grass-Fed Whey Protein Isolate

Ice

**PREPARATION:**

1st version: combine carrot and orange juice and mix them well. The juice is ready to drink.

2nd version: coconut milk can be added in the 1st version. Mix well or put them in a mixer.

3rd version: Place carrot juice, orange juice, coconut milk, protein powder, and ice in a blender and zap it until frothy, icy, and blended. Serve immediately.

**NUTRITION**

Calories: 79kcal | Carbohydrates: 10g | Protein: 8g | Fat: 1g

# LOW FODMAP CREAM OF TOMATO SOUP WITH GRILLED CHEESE CROUTONS

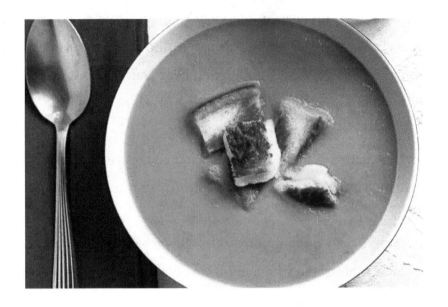

Makes: 3 Servings Prep Time: 15 minutes Cook Time: 25 minutes
Total Time: 40 minutes

At room temperature, sliced very thinly

PREPARATION:

For the Soup: Heat oil over low-medium heat in a large Dutch oven or heavy pot until shimmering. Add scallion greens and sauté until softened but not browned.

Add tomatoes and juice and crush tomatoes with a masher. Add seasonings and bring to a boil.

Adjust heat to a simmer, cover pot, and cook for 15 minutes. Taste and adjust seasoning.

Carefully transfer to blender and purée, or purée right in the pot if you have an immersion blender. You can leave as is, or for a more classic texture, strain through a fine-meshed strainer and return to pot to reheat. Add cream, heat gently, but do not boil. Keep warm.

For the Grilled Cheese Croutons: You make the grilled cheese while the soup is cooking to save time if you want to multitask.

Lay your bread out on your work surface in front of you and spread a tablespoon of mayonnaise on each slice, edge to edge, covering completely.

Place a large nonstick or cast-iron pan on the stove over low heat and add butter. Melt the butter and swirl it around the pan. Place two slices of bread in the pan, mayo side down. Divide cheese between the two pieces of bread and top with remaining bread, mayo side up. Increase heat to low-medium. Cook until the bottom is golden brown, flip, and continue cooking until the second side is equally crispy and golden and cheese is melted.

Pour hot soup into warm bowls. Cut sandwiches into small square "croutons", about 1-inch (2.5 cm) across. Divide croutons amongst bowls and serve immediately.

## NUTRITION

Calories: 524kcal | Carbohydrates: 48g | Protein: 13g | Fat: 47g | Saturated Fat: 2g | Cholesterol: 8mg | Sodium: 744mg | Sugar: 14g

# LOW FODMAP CARAMELIZED PINEAPPLE SAUCE

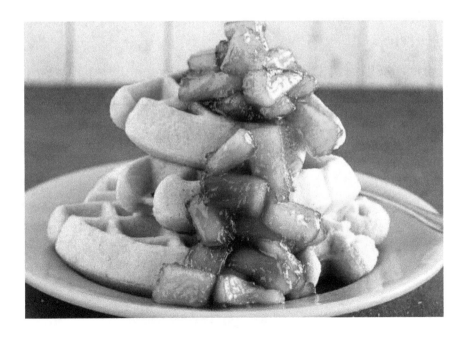

Makes: 8 Servings Prep Time: 5 minutes Cook Time: 10 minutes Total Time: 15 minutes

## INGREDIENTS:

6 tablespoons (85 g) unsalted butter, cut into pieces

½ cup (107 g) firmly packed light brown sugar

4 cups (560 g) fresh pineapple chunks

¾ cup (180 ml) pure maple syrup

## PREPARATION:

Put butter in a pot and melt it. Add brown sugar and cook until sugar gets dissolved. Add pineapples and cook until butter/sugar mixture gets caramelize and toss pineapple well. Add maple syrup and cook all get mixed well. Remove from heat and let it cool. It is ready to eat now.

## NUTRITION

Calories: 189kcal | Carbohydrates: 29g | Protein: 1g | Fat: 8g | Sodium: 2mg | Potassium: 50mg | Fiber: 1g | Sugar: 13g | Calcium: 24mg | Iron: 1mg

# LOW FODMAP RANCH DRESSING

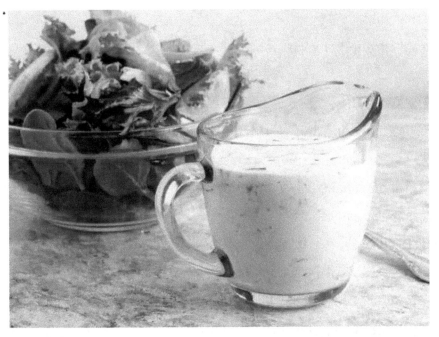

Makes: 4 Servings Prep Time: 10 minutes Total Time: 10 minutes

INGREDIENTS:

½ cup (120 ml) lactose-free whole milk

2 teaspoons freshly squeezed lemon juice

½ cup (113 g) mayonnaise

2 tablespoons finely chopped fresh chives or 2 teaspoons dried chives

1 tablespoon finely chopped fresh dill or 1 teaspoon dried dill

1 tablespoon finely chopped fresh flat-leaf parsley or 1 teaspoon dried parsley

1 tablespoon finely chopped scallions, green parts only

2 teaspoons Garlic-Infused Oil, made with vegetable oil or purchased garlic-flavored vegetable oil

½ teaspoon Dijon mustard

Kosher salt

Freshly ground black pepper

PREPARATION:

Mix lime juice and milk in a jar and let it set aside until it gets thick. Add mayonnaise, scallions, chives, parsley, dill, oil, and mustard. Cover it and shake it well. Add seasonings according to taste. The dressing is ready to use.

NUTRITION

Calories: 235kcal | Carbohydrates: 2g | Protein: 1g | Fat: 25g | Saturated Fat: 3g | Cholesterol: 12mg | Sodium: 195mg | Fiber: 1g | Sugar: 2g | Vitamin A: 19IU | Iron: 1mg

# LOW FODMAP PASTA PRIMAVERA

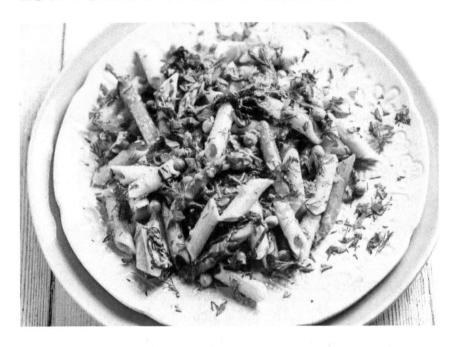

Makes: 6 Servings Prep Time: 10 minutes Cook Time: 15 minutes
Total Time: 25 minutes

**INGREDIENTS:**

2 tablespoons Onion-Infused Oil, made with shallots and olive oil;
extra if needed

1/3 cup (24 g) chopped chives or scallion greens

3 ½ cups (840 ml) water

Kosher salt

12- ounces (340 g) low FODMAP, gluten-free penne, such as Jovial
brand

3 asparagus stalks, trimmed, cut into 2-inch (5 cm) lengths

3- ounces (85 g) fresh baby arugula leaves

3- ounces (85 g) fresh baby spinach leaves

60 grams frozen peas, about 1/3 cup

2 tablespoons unsalted butter

3- ounces (85 g) finely grated Parmesan cheese

2 tablespoons freshly squeezed lemon juice, plus 1 teaspoon finely grated lemon zest

2 tablespoons chopped fresh dill

2 tablespoons chopped fresh tarragon

Freshly ground black pepper

**PREPARATION:**

Add oil to a pan and heat it. Add scallion green until they get soft and brown. Add pasta, water, and a pinch of salt. Stir well and bring it to a boil. After 4 minutes add the asparagus and cook for about 30 seconds, then stir the arugula and spinach into the pasta and water. Re-cover the pot. Keep cooking until pasta gets tender. Do not let water vanished. Add peas and cook for 30 seconds. Remove from heat and add lemon zest, lime juice, and parmesan and stir well. It is ready to use.

**NUTRITION**

Calories: 325kcal | Carbohydrates: 44g | Protein: 10g | Fat: 13g | Sodium: 139mg | Fiber: 2g | Calcium: 4mg

# LOW FODMAP GRATED CARROT SALAD

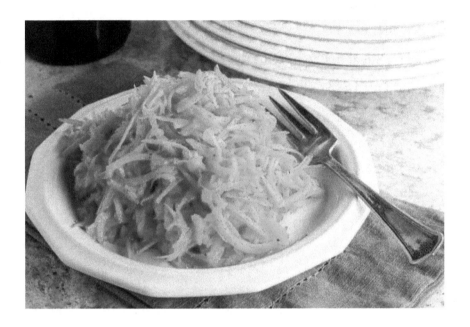

Makes: 6 Servings Prep Time: 10 minutes Total Time: 10 minutes

INGREDIENTS:

1- Pound (455 g) carrots, trimmed and peeled, shredded

1 fresh large heavy lemon, halved, pitted

2 to 4 tablespoons (2 tablespoons to 60 ml) extra-virgin olive oil, divided

Kosher salt

Freshly ground black pepper

PREPARATION:

Peel and grate carrots. Add a little amount of oil and lime juice and toss well. Add seasonings according to your taste. Mix well and you are set to eat.

NUTRITION

Calories: 73kcal | Carbohydrates: 7g | Protein: 1g | Fat: 5g | Saturated Fat: 1g | Sodium: 1mg | Fiber: 2g | Sugar: 3g

# NO FODMAP FRUIT SALAD

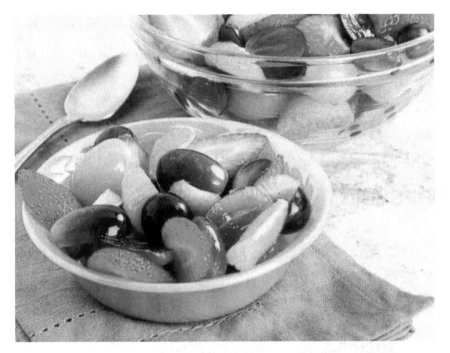

Makes: 6 Servings Prep Time: 10 minutes Total Time: 10 minutes

**INGREDIENTS:**

1- Pound (455 g) strawberries

4 clementines; (or 2 navel oranges)

2 cups (300 g) grapes; I like a mixture of seedless black, green and red

**PREPARATION:**

Hull the strawberries, then halve or quarter. Peel and section the clementines. Halve the grapes.

Just mix all fruits well and your fruit salad is ready to eat.

**NUTRITION**

Calories: 102kcal | Carbohydrates: 26g | Protein: 1g | Fat: 1g | Saturated Fat: 1g | Sodium: 3mg | Potassium: 354mg | Fiber: 3g | Sugar: 20g | Vitamin A: 61IU | Vitamin C: 71mg | Calcium: 35mg | Iron: 1mg

# NO FODMAP MALT VINEGAR SALAD DRESSING

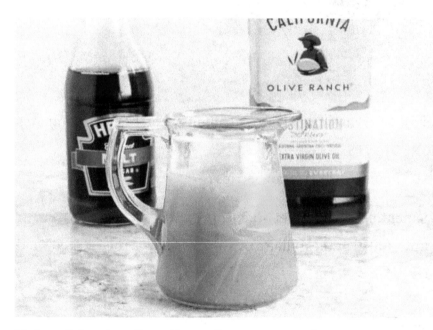

Makes: 8 Servings Prep Time: 5 minutes Total Time: 5 minutes

**INGREDIENTS:**

¾ cup (180 ml) extra virgin olive oil

1/3 cup (75 ml) malt vinegar

Kosher salt

Freshly ground black pepper

**PREPARATION:**

Mix and shake vinegar and oil together in a jar. Add salt and pepper according to taste and mix well. The dressing is ready to use or you can place it in a refrigerator.

**NUTRITION**

Calories: 198kcal | Carbohydrates: 1g | Fat: 22g | Saturated Fat: 3g | Sodium: 1mg | Sugar: 1g | Iron: 1mg

# NO FODMAP VEGETABLE SALAD

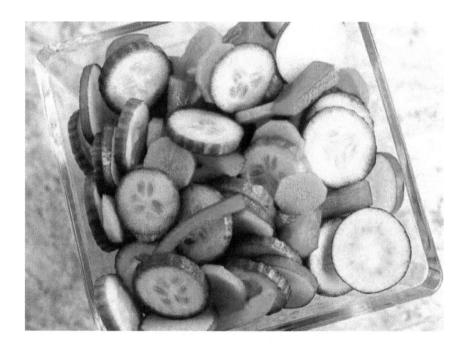

Makes: 4 Servings Prep Time: 5 minutes Total Time: 5 minutes

INGREDIENTS:

6 red radishes, trimmed, sliced crosswise into discs

2 medium carrots, trimmed, peeled, and cut crosswise into discs

2 small Persian cucumbers or half an English hothouse cucumber, cut crosswise into discs

1 red bell pepper, cored and cut into strips

Kosher salt; optional

Freshly ground black pepper; optional

Olive oil; optional

No FODMAP Malt Vinegar Salad Dressing

**PREPARATION:**

Simply toss the vegetables together and the salad is ready to enjoy. Add seasonings including salt and pepper in the required amount and enjoy the salad. A little vinegar can be added.

**NUTRITION**

Calories: 32kcal | Carbohydrates: 6g | Protein: 1g | Fat: 1g | Fiber: 2g | Sugar: 3g

# LOW FODMAP EGGPLANT DIP

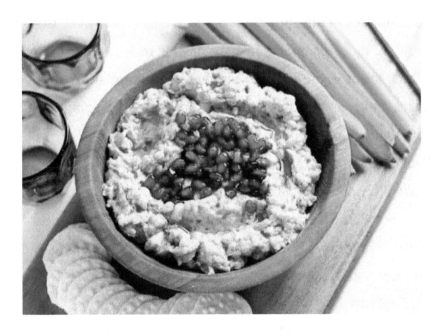

Makes: 8 Servings Prep Time: 10 minutes Cook Time: 1 hour Total Time: 1 hour 10 minutes

**INGREDIENTS:**

2, large globe eggplants, about 1 ½ pounds/680 g each, washed and dried

¼ cup (60 ml) tahini

1 tablespoon freshly squeezed lemon juice, or to taste

Kosher salt

Garlic-Infused Olive Oil

Pomegranate seeds; optional

**PREPARATION:**

Position rack in the upper part of the oven. Preheat oven to 400°F (200°C). Place eggplant directly on the rack (or on a rimmed baking sheet if you want to prevent any potential drips in your oven) and roast for about an hour or until the eggplant is super soft, tender, and wrinkly. Remove and cool.

Peel eggplant and take out the flesh. Mash the flesh in a bowl or make a puree by blending it in a blender. Add tahini and lemon juice according to taste. Taste and add salt and pepper according to need. Take it in a bowl. Add oil and garnish it with pomegranate seeds. It is all set to use.

**NUTRITION**

Calories: 78kcal | Carbohydrates: 10g | Protein: 3g | Fat: 4g | Saturated Fat: 1g | Sodium: 3mg | Potassium: 34mg | Fiber: 5g | Sugar: 3g | Vitamin C: 1mg | Calcium: 10mg | Iron: 1mg

# LOW FODMAP CARROT CONSOMMÉ

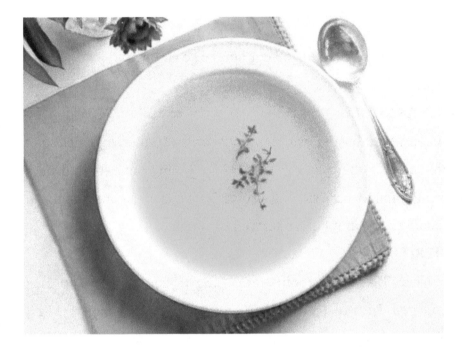

Makes: 8 Servings Prep Time: 10 minutes Cook Time: 3 hours
Total Time: 3 hours 10 minutes

**INGREDIENTS:**

3 quarts (2.8 L ) water

4- pounds (1.8 kg) carrots, trimmed, peeled, and cut into large chunks

1 cup (72 g) chopped leeks, green parts only

2- Inches (5 cm) fresh ginger, peeled and cut in half lengthwise

5 black peppercorns

2 whole cloves

2 bay leaves

2 sprigs fresh thyme

1 celery stalk, trimmed and cut into large chunks

Kosher salt

**PREPARATION:**

Add all vegetables in water to a pot. Cook them on high heat and then simmer them for 3 hours. After getting done, pass it on a strainer and discard the vegetables. Taste the consomme and add seasonings. Heat it before serving.

**NUTRITION**

Calories: 97kcal | Carbohydrates: 23g | Protein: 3g | Fat: 1g | Saturated Fat: 1g | Sodium: 18mg | Fiber: 7g | Sugar: 11g | Calcium: 11mg

# EASY STOVETOP LOW FODMAP MAC AND CHEESE

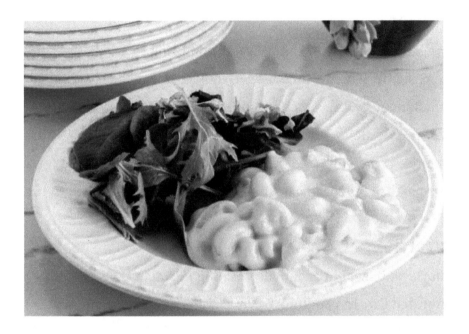

Makes: 6 Servings Prep Time: 10 minutes Cook Time: 15 minutes Total Time: 25 minutes

**INGREDIENTS:**

12- ounces (340 g) low FODMAP, gluten-free elbow pasta, such as Jovial brand

½ cup (1 stick; 113 g) unsalted butter, cut into pieces

½ cup (73 g) low FODMAP, gluten-free all-purpose flour

1 ¼ teaspoon dry, powdered mustard

1 teaspoon kosher salt

½ teaspoon white pepper

3 cups (720 ml) lactose-free whole milk, at room temperature

8- ounces (225 g) sharp cheddar cheese, shredded; I like using orange colored

**PREPARATION:**

Bring a large pot with salted water and bring to a boil and cook the pasta till al dente; do not over-cook. Drain and set aside.

Simultaneously, take another pot and add butter to it. Heat it and melt it. Add flour, salt, mustard, and pepper. Cook it for 1 to 2 minutes. Gradually add milk and cook until the sauce gets thickened. Remove from heat and add pasta and fold it well. Serve it.

**NUTRITION**

Calories: 601kcal | Carbohydrates: 58g | Protein: 19g | Fat: 33g | Saturated Fat: 1g | Sodium: 619mg | Fiber: 2g | Sugar: 6g

# LOW FODMAP JAPANESE PICKLES

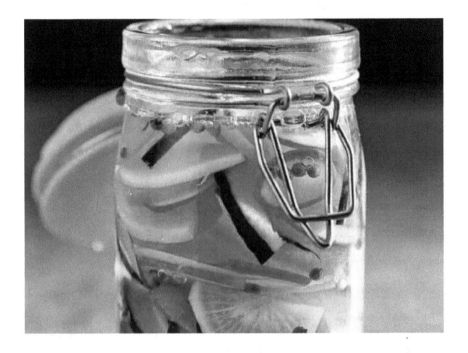

Makes: 6 Servings Prep Time: 5 minutes Cook Time: 2 minutes

Cooking Time: 30 minutes Total Time: 37 minutes

**INGREDIENTS:**

Pickling Liquor:

1 teaspoon cilantro seeds

1 teaspoon cumin seeds

¼ cup (60 ml) water

Juice of 1 lime

1 to 2 tablespoons caster sugar

1 teaspoon of sea salt

Vegetables:

½ standard cucumber finely sliced, seeds removed

3- Ounces (55 g) daikon, finely sliced

2- Ounces (55 g) salad radishes, finely sliced

½ cup (120 ml) rice or white vinegar

**PREPARATION:**

Place a non-stick pan over heat and add cilantro and cumin seeds and cook for 1 to 2 minutes.

Add all remaining pickle ingredients and cook. Once the sugar and salt get dissolved remove the pan from heat. Let it cool. Add vegetables and vinegar and let it pickle. Store it in an airtight jar.

**NUTRITION**

Calories: 29kcal | Carbohydrates: 6g | Protein: 1g | Fat: 1g | Saturated Fat: 1g | Sodium: 392mg | Potassium: 6mg | Fiber: 1g | Sugar: 4g | Calcium: 3mg | Iron: 1mg

# LOW FODMAP LEMON GRANITA

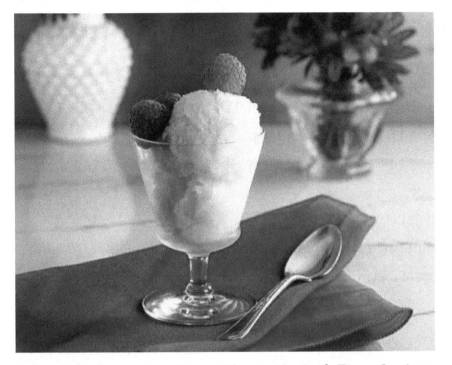

Makes: 8 Servings Prep Time: 15 minutes Cook Time: 3 minutes

Chilling Time: 4 hours Total Time: 4 hours 18 minutes

**INGREDIENTS:**

2 ½ cups (600 ml) water, divided

1 cup (198 g) sugar

1 cup (240 ml) freshly squeezed lemon juice

1 ½ teaspoon finely grated lemon zest

Optional: pomegranate seeds, or fresh firm raspberries

**PREPARATION:**

Combine half of the water and sugar in a medium saucepan. Stir to wet the sugar. Place over medium heat and bring to a simmer. Cook until the sugar dissolves, swirling the pot once or twice. Remove from the heat, cool to room temperature, and stir in the remaining water, lemon juice, and zest. Pour into an 8-inch (20 cm) or 9-inch (23 cm) metal pan.

Freeze for 45 minutes or until it starts getting freeze. Take a fork and take out the frozen parts other than the liquid part. Check again and again and take out all of the crystals. This granita is ready to use.

**NUTRITION**

Calories: 122kcal | Carbohydrates: 32g | Protein: 1g | Sodium: 4mg | Fiber: 1g | Sugar: 30g | Calcium: 2mg

# GARLICKY LOW FODMAP SAUTÉED KALE WITH CHESTNUTS

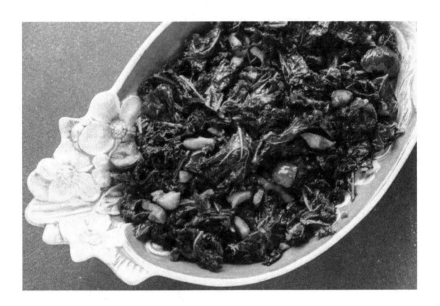

Makes: 10 Servings Prep Time: 5 minutes Cook Time: 5 minutes
Total Time: 10 minutes

**INGREDIENTS:**

¼ cup (60 ml) Garlic-Infused Oil, made with olive oil or purchased
equivalent

20- ounces (570 g) curly kale, stemmed and chopped or torn into
bite-sized pieces

6- ounces (170 g) cooked chestnuts, chopped

2 tablespoons orange juice

Kosher salt

Freshly ground black pepper

**PREPARATION:**

Heat oil on medium heat and add kale into it. Cook until they are soft and crisp. Add orange juice and nuts. Season it with salt and pepper according to need. It is ready to serve.

**NUTRITION**

Calories: 118kcal | Carbohydrates: 32g | Protein: 2g | Fat: 6g | Saturated Fat: 1g | Sodium: 1mg | Potassium: 7mg | Fiber: 5g | Sugar: 1g | Vitamin A: 7IU | Vitamin C: 2mg

# VEGAN NO FODMAP ROOT VEGETABLE SOUP

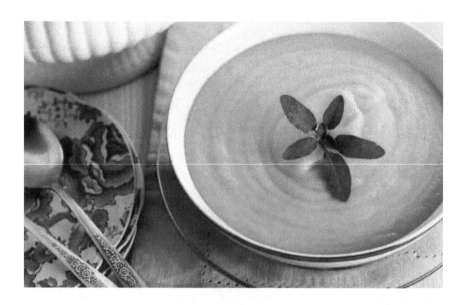

Makes: 4 Servings Prep Time: 5 minutes Cook Time: 30 minutes Total Time: 35 minutes

**INGREDIENTS:**

3 tablespoons Low FODMAP Garlic-Infused Oil, made with olive oil or purchased the equivalent

1 cup (64 g) roughly chopped scallions, green parts only

4 medium carrots, trimmed, peeled, and cut into chunks

4 medium parsnips, trimmed, peeled, and cut into chunks

1- Pound (455 g) Yukon Gold potatoes, peeled and cut into chunks

3 cups (720 ml) Low FODMAP Vegetable Broth

1 cup (240 ml) unsweetened almond milk

Kosher salt

Freshly ground black pepper

Garnish – fresh parsley, sage, thyme, or nothing at all!

**PREPARATION:**

Heat oil on the Dutch oven and add scallions. Add carrots, parsnips, potatoes, and broth. The broth must be covered. Cook it for 20 minutes.

Make a puree of soup in a blender. If there is no blender then transfer the soup to a blender in batches and blend until smooth. Take care as the soup is hot; follow your blender manufacturer's instructions.

Put almond milk and blend to form a smooth paste. Taste it and then add seasonings including salt and pepper. Garnish it with fresh herbs and serve.

**NUTRITION**

Calories: 289kcal | Carbohydrates: 45g | Protein: 6g | Fat: 11g | Saturated Fat: 1g | Sodium: 11mg | Potassium: 468mg | Fiber: 5g | Sugar: 8g | Vitamin C: 13mg | Calcium: 34mg | Iron: 4mg

# LOW FODMAP BRUSSELS SPROUTS SALAD

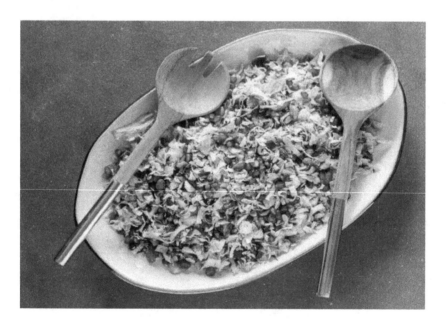

Makes: 8 Servings Prep Time: 10 minutes Total Time: 10 minutes

**INGREDIENTS:**

Salad:

10- ounces (280 g) fresh Brussels sprouts, trimmed to equal 8-ounces (225 g) and shredded

1 large head Romaine lettuce, cored and shredded, (about 5 to 6-ounces)

½ cup (69 g) toasted whole smoked almonds, chopped

½ cup (87 g) pomegranate seeds

¼ cup (8 g) chopped fresh flat-leaf parsley

Dressing:

1/3 cup (75 ml) extra virgin olive oil

1/3 cup (75 ml) freshly squeezed lemon juice

2 teaspoons Dijon mustard

2 teaspoons maple syrup; optional

Kosher salt

Freshly ground black pepper

Shaved Parmesan; optional

**PREPARATION:**

Toss and mix all vegetables and make a salad.

Add lemon juice, oil, maple syrup, and mustard in a jar and shake well. Add salt and pepper and put over salad. Salad is ready to serve.

**NUTRITION**

Calories: 148kcal | Carbohydrates: 8g | Protein: 3g | Fat: 13g |
Saturated Fat: 1g | Sodium: 15mg | Potassium: 35mg | Fiber: 1g |
Sugar: 3g | Vitamin C: 2mg | Calcium: 3mg | Iron: 1mg

# OVEN-BAKED LOW FODMAP PARSNIP FRIES

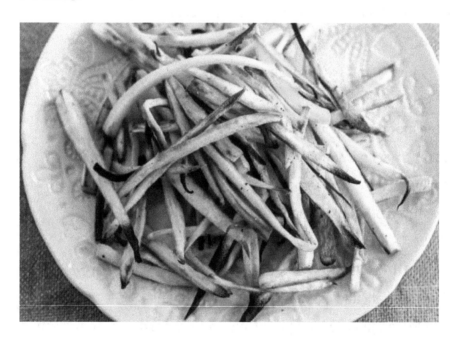

Makes: 4 Servings Prep Time: 5 minutes Cook Time: 30 minutes
Total Time: 35 minutes

**INGREDIENTS:**

1- Pound (455 g) parsnips, (about 4 medium parsnips)

2 tablespoons extra virgin olive oil

Kosher salt

Freshly ground black pepper

PREPARATION:

Position rack at the top of the oven. Preheat oven to 450°F (230°C).

Peel and cut parsnips. Discard the stem part and cut into fries shape. Spread parsnips on a baking tray and put oil, salt, and pepper. Toss well so that there is even coating.

Bake them for 15 minutes then turn them and again roast for 15 minutes. When they are done they are ready to serve.

**NUTRITION**

Calories: 147kcal | Carbohydrates: 20g | Protein: 1g | Fat: 7g | Saturated Fat: 1g | Sodium: 11mg | Potassium: 425mg | Fiber: 6g | Sugar: 5g | Vitamin C: 19mg | Calcium: 41mg | Iron: 1mg

# LOW FODMAP BERRY CHIA JELLY

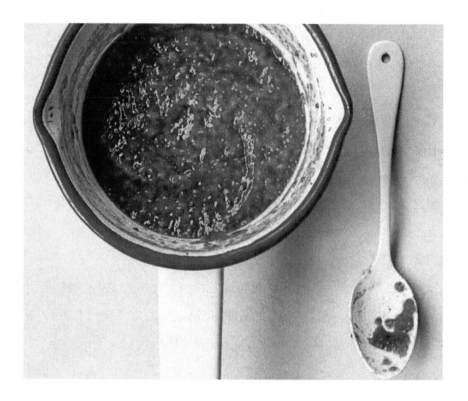

Makes: 8 Servings Prep Time: 5 minutes Cook Time: 20 minutes

Total Time: 25 minutes

**INGREDIENTS:**

About 1 cup (150 g) hulled strawberries

2 tablespoons chia seeds

2 tablespoons pure maple syrup

¼ cup (60 ml) water

**PREPARATION:**

Put all ingredients in a blender and blend them to make a smooth paste. Transfer this paste to a pot and bring it to a boil. Reduce the heat and cook for 20 minutes.

Let the jelly cool and put it in an airtight container and serve it.

**NUTRITION**

Calories: 34kcal | Carbohydrates: 6g | Protein: 1g | Fat: 1g | Saturated Fat: 1g | Sodium: 1mg | Potassium: 23mg | Fiber: 1g | Sugar: 4g | Calcium: 24mg | Iron: 1mg

# LOW FODMAP LENTIL SALAD WITH GREENS & YOGURT

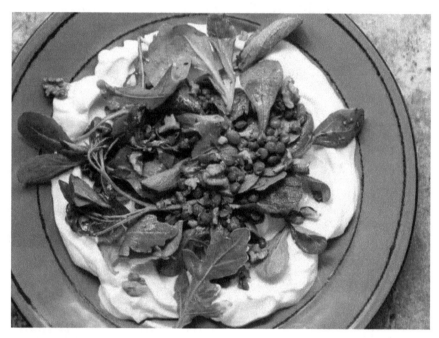

Makes: 6 Servings Prep Time: 10 minutes Total Time: 10 minutes

**INGREDIENTS:**

3 tablespoons Garlic-Infused Oil, made with olive oil or purchased equivalent, divided

1/3 cup (45 g) walnut halves, chopped

1 teaspoon cumin seed

1 cup (255 g) thick lactose-free plain yogurt, such as Siggi's

Kosher salt

Freshly ground black pepper

1- Ounce (30 g) baby arugula

1- Ounce (30 g) baby lettuces

1 cup (164 g) well-drained canned green (brown) lentils

2 tablespoons freshly squeezed lemon juice

**PREPARATION:**

Heat 1 tablespoon of the oil in a nonstick skillet over low-medium heat and add the walnuts and the cumin seed. Toss frequently and cook just until lightly toasted and the cumin smells fragrant. Remove from heat and set aside.

Spread the thick yogurt on your serving platter to about 1/3-inch (8 m thickness. Salt and pepper lightly.

Add lettuces, arugula, and lentils in a bowl. Add nuts and cumin seeds along with any oil. Add seasonings to this mixture. Do not add a lot of dressing over salad. Add lentils and greens to the top of the salad and serve.

**NUTRITION**

Calories: 166kcal | Carbohydrates: 11g | Protein: 6g | Fat: 12g | Saturated Fat: 1g | Sodium: 2mg | Potassium: 23mg | Fiber: 3g | Sugar: 3g | Vitamin A: 112IU | Vitamin C: 1mg | Calcium: 11mg | Iron: 1mg

# LOW FODMAP CHEDDAR CHEESE

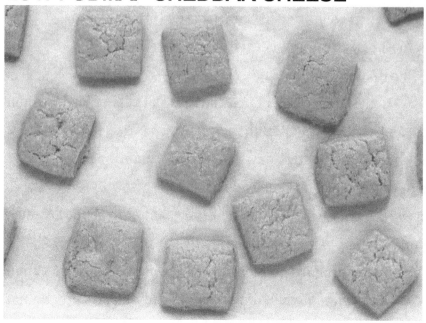

Makes: 24 Servings Prep Time: 10 minutes Cook Time: 15 minutes
Chilling: 1 hour Total Time: 1 hour 25 minutes

INGREDIENTS:

- 1- Pound (455 g) sharp or extra-sharp cheddar, (we like orange-colored cheddar)

1 cup (113 g; 2 sticks) unsalted butter, at room temperature, cut into pieces

1 large egg yolk

2 teaspoons Dijon mustard

2 teaspoons salt

¼ teaspoon cayenne

1 ¾ cups (254 g) all-purpose gluten-free low FODMAP flour, such as Bob's Red Mill 1 to 1 Gluten-Free Baking Flour, plus additional for dusting

**PREPARATION:**

Grate cheese in a food processor using a grater disc (either coarse or fine). Switch to the multi-purpose blade. Add butter and yolk and process until smooth. Add remaining ingredients and pulse until just combined. Scrape soft dough onto a large piece of plastic, wrap well, flatten slightly and refrigerate at least 1 hour or overnight.

Place racks in upper and lower thirds of the oven and preheat oven to 350°F (180°C). Line 2 baking sheet pans with parchment paper.

Roll out dough on a lightly floured surface to 1/8-inch (3 thickness. If the dough is giving you any problems, simply roll out in-between two pieces of parchment. Cut the rolled out dough into a grid to create small, 1-inch (2.5 square crackers. Place on prepared pans evenly spaced apart.

Bake for about 12 to 15 min; adjust the time for different sized crackers. The crackers should be a little puffed, beginning to color and there might be a little cheese and butter oozing out and bubbling slightly along the bottom edges.

Cool pan completely on rack. Crackers may be stored for up to 4 days at room temperature in airtight containers.

NUTRITION

Calories: 183kcal | Carbohydrates: 9g | Protein: 5g | Fat: 14g | Saturated Fat: 1g | Sodium: 314mg | Fiber: 1g | Sugar: 1g | Vitamin A: 9IU

# LOW FODMAP OVERNIGHT OATS & CHIA

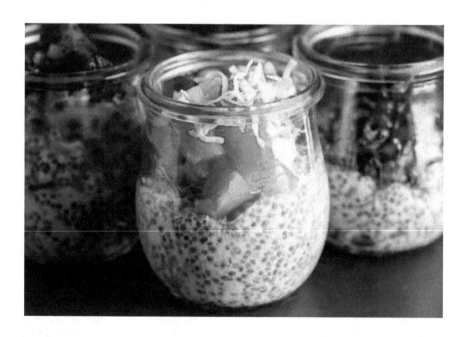

Makes: 6 Servings Prep Time: 10 minutes Chilling Time 8 hours Total Time: 8 hours 10 minutes

**INGREDIENTS:**

1 1/3 cups (315 ml) unsweetened almond milk

1 cup (99 g) old-fashioned rolled oats; do not use quick or instant; use gluten-free if following a gluten-free diet

3 tablespoons chia seeds

1 to 2 tablespoons maple syrup; optional

PREPARATION:

Add all ingredients to a jar. Shake well so that all ingredients can be mixed completely. After getting done place it in the refrigerator for the whole night. Scoop out and serve it.

NUTRITION

Calories: 194kcal | Carbohydrates: 31g | Protein: 6g | Fat: 4g | Saturated Fat: 1g | Sodium: 4mg | Potassium: 175mg | Fiber: 6g | Sugar: 2g | Calcium: 62mg | Iron: 2.1mg

# LOW FODMAP MINT CHUTNEY

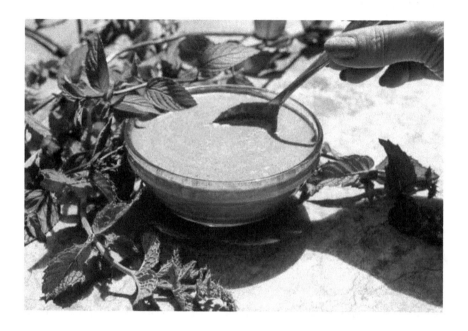

Makes: 8 Servings Prep Time: 5 minutes Total Time: 5 minutes

INGREDIENTS:

¼ cup (60 ml) to 6 tablespoons (90 ml) freshly squeezed lemon juice

2 tablespoons Garlic-Infused Oil, made with vegetable oil or purchased the equivalent

1 cup (26 g) firmly packed fresh mint leaves, (or cilantro leaves, for that variation

1 cup (64 g) roughly chopped scallions, green parts only

2 green Serrano chiles, stemmed and seeded

2 teaspoons sugar

1 teaspoon low FODMAP Garam Masala

1 teaspoon kosher salt

PREPARATION:

Put lemon juice, oil, mint, chiles, sugar, scallions, salt, and garam masala in a blender. Blend until a smooth puree is formed. Green chutney is ready to serve.

NUTRITION

Calories: 40kcal | Carbohydrates: 2g | Protein: 1g | Fat: 4g | Sodium: 291mg | Fiber: 1g | Sugar: 1g

# LOW FODMAP CANTALOUPE LIME POPSICLES

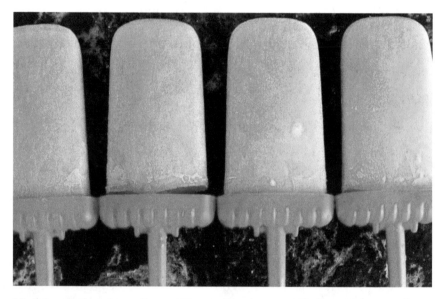

Makes: 8 Servings Prep Time: 5 minutes Chilling Time 8 hours
Total Time: 8 hours 5 minutes

INGREDIENTS:

¾ cup (180 ml) water

1/3 cup (65 g) sugar

20- ounces (570 g) chunks of ripe orange cantaloupe

1 tablespoon plus 1 teaspoon freshly squeezed lime juice

PREPARATION:

Mix water and sugar both overheat. Cook it until the sugar gets dissolved. When it is done remove the pan from heat and let it cool.

Place cantaloupe, lime juice, and cooled sugar syrup into blender carafe, cover, and blend until super smooth and blended. Put this mixture in the popsicle mold evenly. Add popsicles stick into it. Freeze it overnight and serve it.

NUTRITION

Calories: 62kcal | Carbohydrates: 16g | Protein: 1g | Fat: 1g | Sodium: 1mg | Fiber: 1g | Sugar: 15g

# LOW FODMAP LIME CHEESECAKE DIP

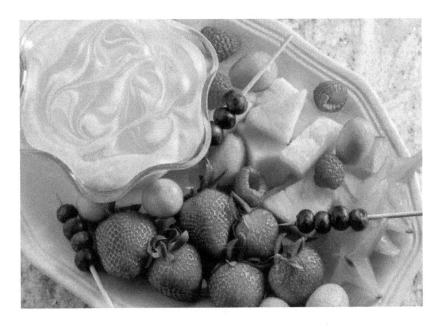

Makes: 8 Servings Prep Time: 10 minutes Total Time: 10 minutes

INGREDIENTS:

8- ounce (225 g) lactose-free cream cheese such as Green Valley Creamery brand

¼ cup (60 g) lactose-free sour cream

¼ cup (76 g) plus 2 tablespoons lime curd, divided

Low FODMAP fruit, such as strawberries, pineapple chunks, carambola, grapes, blueberries threaded onto skewers, etc.

Low FODMAP cookies or pretzels

PREPARATION:

Gently mix sour cream, lime curd, and cream cheese until they are blended well. Put this into a serving platter. Add remaining lime curd on top. Cheesecake dips are ready to serve.

NUTRITION

Calories: 156kcal | Carbohydrates: 6g | Protein: 2g | Fat: 14g | Sugar: 4g | Vitamin A: 125IU | Calcium: 5mg

# LOW FODMAP PARSLEY PESTO

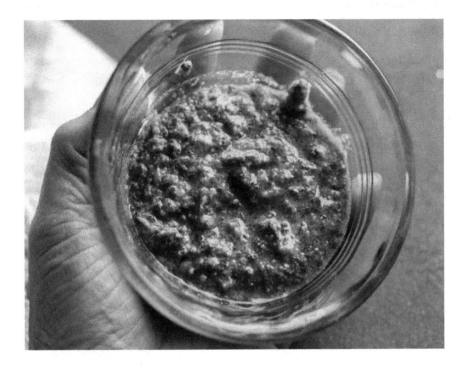

Makes: 8 Servings Prep Time: 10 minutes Total Time: 10 minutes

INGREDIENTS:

¾ cup (180 ml) Garlic-Infused Oil, made with olive oil or purchased equivalent, divided

2 tablespoons lemon juice

2 cups (about 40 g) lightly packed washed and dried fresh flat-leaf parsley leaves

¼ cup (34 g) lightly toasted pine nuts

Kosher salt

Freshly ground black pepper

Water, if needed

Add garlic-infused oil, lemon juice, parsley leaves, and pine nuts in a blender. Blend it well to form a smooth paste. Add salt and pepper according to taste. If pesto is thick then add water. Pesto is ready to use.

NUTRITION

Calories: 223kcal | Carbohydrates: 1g | Fat: 23g | Vitamin C: 1.5mg

# LOW FODMAP POPPY SEED DRESSING

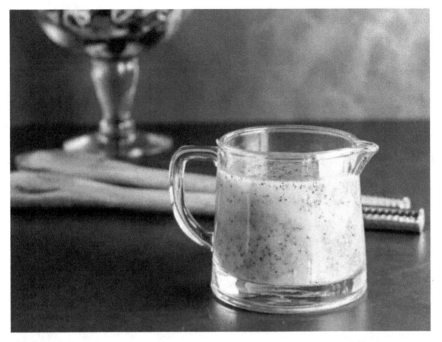

Makes: 6 Servings Prep Time: 5 minutes Total Time: 5 minutes

INGREDIENTS:

½ cup ( 120 ml) neutral-flavored vegetable oil

¼ cup (60 ml) apple cider vinegar or red wine vinegar (see Tips)

1 ½ tablespoons poppy seeds

1 tablespoon very finely minced scallions, green parts only; optional

1 tablespoon sugar (or honey; see Tips)

1 teaspoon Dijon mustard

Kosher salt

PREPARATION:

Put all ingredients along with oil and mustard in a jar. Shake it well so that all ingredients can be mixed. Taste it and add seasonings. It is ready to use.

NUTRITION

Calories: 183kcal | Carbohydrates: 3g | Protein: 1g | Fat: 18g | Saturated Fat: 1g | Sodium: 10mg | Potassium: 16mg | Fiber: 1g | Sugar: 2g | Calcium: 32mg | Iron: 0.2mg

# LOW FODMAP BLUEBERRY LIMEADE

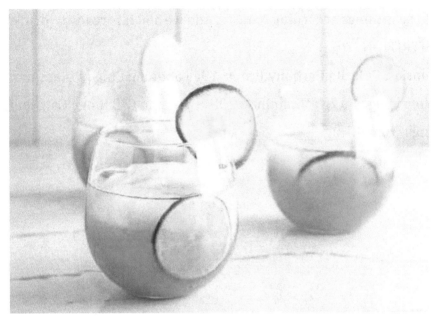

Makes: 6 Servings Prep Time: 10 minutes Total Time: 10 minutes

INGREDIENTS:

1 cup (160 g) blueberries

1/3 cup (65 g) sugar, plus more if needed

4 cups (960 ml) water

6 tablespoons (90 ml) freshly squeezed lime juice

Ice cubes

Lime slices or wedges as a garnish; optional

PREPARATION:

Put blueberries in a mixing bowl along with sugar. Mash it with a potato masher and allow it to set. Pass it through a strainer and get the desired juice. Mix the juice with water and lime juice and add seasonings according to taste. Add ice and it is ready to drink.

NUTRITION

Calories: 76kcal | Carbohydrates: 19g | Sodium: 8mg | Potassium: 30mg | Sugar: 17g | Vitamin A: 20IU | Vitamin C: 3.8mg | Calcium: 7mg | Iron: 0.1mg

# LOW FODMAP APPLE & WALNUT CHAROSET

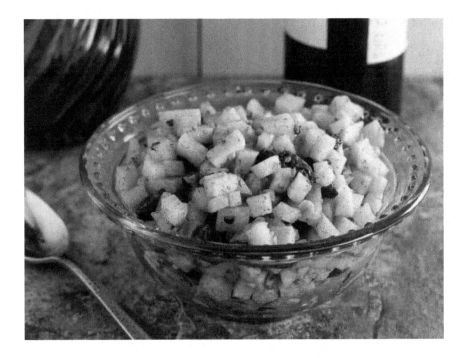

Makes: 12 Servings Prep Time: 10 minutes Total Time: 10 minutes

INGREDIENTS:

1- Pound (455 g) jicama, peeled and finely diced

4 ¼ ounces (120 g) peeled and cored finely diced Pink Lady apple

¾ cup (75 g) toasted walnut halves, finely chopped

½ cup (83 g) raisins

1 ½ tablespoon red wine or cranberry juice

1 tablespoon honey

1 teaspoon firmly packed light brown sugar

½ teaspoon cinnamon

Pinch teaspoon cloves

Pinch teaspoon nutmeg

PREPARATION:

Take out a medium mixing bowl. Add all the required ingredients to it. Mix all ingredients well so that they combine well. Put this into the refrigerator for 1 hour and then it is set to use.

NUTRITION

Calories: 104kcal | Carbohydrates: 15g | Protein: 2g | Fat: 5g | Saturated Fat: 1g | Sodium: 3mg | Potassium: 81mg | Fiber: 3g | Sugar: 2g | Vitamin C: 0.5mg | Calcium: 3mg | Iron: 0.3mg

# LOW FODMAP GRAPEFRUIT & GREENS SALAD WITH CANDIED PECANS

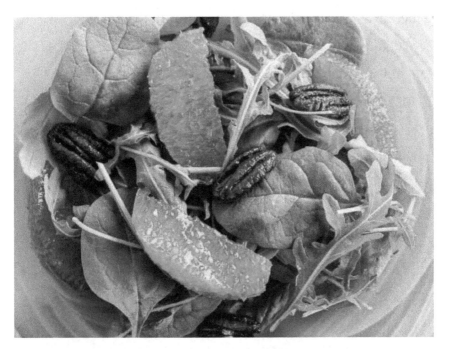

Makes: 8 servings Prep Time: 10 minutes Total Time: 10 minutes

INGREDIENTS:

1 medium grapefruit

2 ounces (40 g) arugula, (about 2 cups, lightly packed)

2 ounces (40 g) baby spinach, (about 2 cups, lightly packed)

½ cup (55 g) Candied Pecans or Candied Spiced Pecans

Red Wine Vinaigrette

PREPARATION:

Prepare grapefruit by peeling it and cutting it downwards on a cutting board. Remove the end stem and the top end of the fruit. Use a knife to loosen wedges of grapefruit by cutting in-between the membranes, releasing the segments into the bowl.

Mix arugula and spinach in the bowl along with nuts. Dress the salad and serve it.

NUTRITION

Calories: 93kcal | Carbohydrates: 5g | Protein: 2g | Fat: 10g | Saturated Fat: 1g | Sodium: 2mg | Potassium: 26mg | Fiber: 1g | Sugar: 2g | Vitamin A: 170IU | Vitamin C: 1.1mg | Calcium: 11mg | Iron: 0.1mg

# LOW FODMAP ORANGE MARMALADE BBQ SAUCE

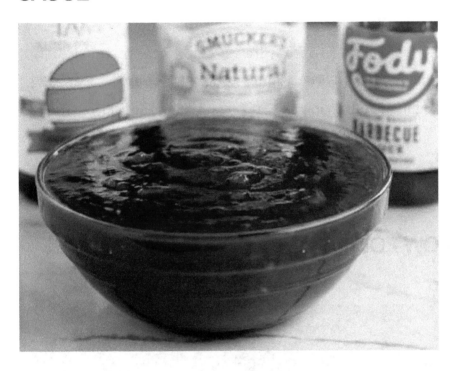

Makes: 16 Servings Prep Time: 5 minutes Total Time: 5 minutes

INGREDIENTS:

1 cup (240 ml) low FODMAP BBQ Sauce

1 cup (304 g) orange marmalade

¼ cup (60 ml) low sodium soy sauce

PREPARATION:

Whish BBQ sauce, orange marmalade, and soy sauce together. This is ready to use immediately or it can be stored in the refrigerator.

NUTRITION

Calories: 56kcal | Carbohydrates: 15g | Protein: 1g | Fat: 1g | Sodium: 179mg | Potassium: 12mg | Fiber: 1g | Sugar: 13g | Vitamin A: 10IU | Vitamin C: 0.7mg | Calcium: 6mg | Iron: 0.1mg

# LOW FODMAP CBD HOT FUDGE SAUCE

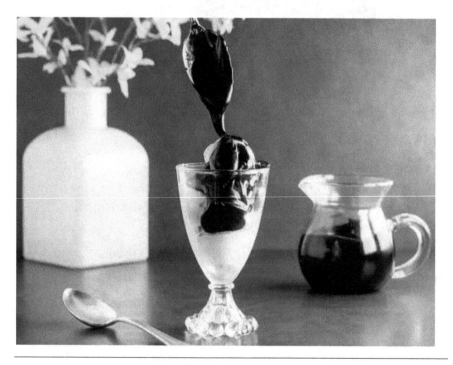

Makes: 12 Servings Prep Time: 5 minutes Cook Time: 5 minutes

Total Time: 10 minutes

INGREDIENTS:

½ cup (120 ml) plus 2 tablespoons lactose-free heavy cream

3 tablespoon unsalted butter, cut into pieces

1/3 cup (65 g) sugar

1/3 cup (71 g) firmly packed light brown sugar

½ cup (43 g) sifted Dutch-processed cocoa

Pinch salt

1 ½ teaspoon CBD hemp oil, such as Elixinol Hemp Extract

PREPARATION:

Cook butter and cream in a pan until butter is melted. Add sugar
and brown sugar to it. Whish well until sugar dissolves. Add cocoa
and salt and whisk until a smooth and shiny paste is formed. Let
it cool now and then it is ready to use.

NUTRITION

Calories: 117kcal | Carbohydrates: 14g | Protein: 1g | Fat: 6g |
Sodium: 1mg | Fiber: 1g | Sugar: 12g

# LOW FODMAP CREAM CHEESE FROSTING

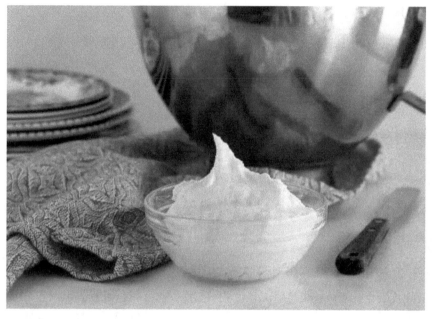

Makes: 12 Servings Prep Time: 5 minutes Total Time: 5 minutes

INGREDIENTS:

6 tablespoons (¾ stick; 85 g) unsalted butter, at room temperature, cut into pieces

3 cups (270 g) sifted confectioners' sugar

½ cup (113 g) Green Valley Creamery lactose-free cream cheese

2 teaspoons lemon juice, preferably freshly squeezed

PREPARATION:

Beat butter in a large bowl with an electric beater for 2 minutes or until it gets smooth. Add cream, sugar, cheese, and lemon juice and beat on low speed. When frosting comes together then increase the speed of the beater and beat for about 3 minutes. The frosting is all set to use.

NUTRITION

Calories: 220kcal | Carbohydrates: 26g | Protein: 1g | Fat: 13g | Sodium: 1mg | Sugar: 23g | Vitamin C: 0.3mg | Calcium: 3mg

# LOW FODMAP GREENS SALAD WITH RADISHES & PEAS

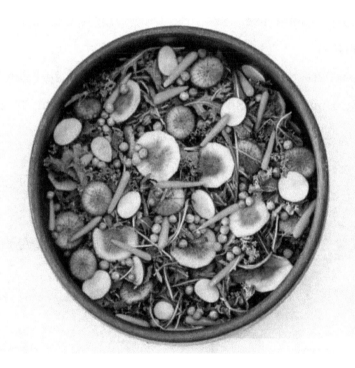

Makes: 8 Servings Prep Time: 10 minutes Total Time: 10 minutes

INGREDIENTS:

Salad:

- 3- Ounces (115 g) cleaned and steamed curly kale, torn into small pieces
- 2- Ounces (55 g) arugula

1- Ounce (30 g) carrots; use you can use tiny, baby carrots as we show here, or cut 1 or 2 medium carrots into rounds or dice

1 medium purple daikon radish, scrubbed or peeled and thinly sliced

1 medium watermelon radish, scrubbed or peeled and thinly sliced

2 red radishes, scrubbed and thinly sliced

¼ cup (38 g) frozen peas, defrosted

Your Choice of Low FODMAP Vinaigrette, such as our Red Wine Vinaigrette

Options:

½ cup (46 g) rinsed and drained canned lentils

2- Ounces 55 g feta, cubed

PREPARATION:

It is a simple and quick recipe. You need to mix and toss all vegetables together. You can add lentils. The salad is ready to use. You can cover it or put it in the refrigerator.

NUTRITION

Calories: 60kcal | Carbohydrates: 8g | Protein: 4g | Fat: 2g | Saturated Fat: 1g | Sodium: 2mg | Potassium: 156mg | Fiber: 3g | Sugar: 2g | Vitamin A: 170IU | Vitamin C: 1.3mg | Calcium: 14mg | Iron: 0.6mg

# LOW FODMAP SPARKLING RHUBARB COCKTAIL

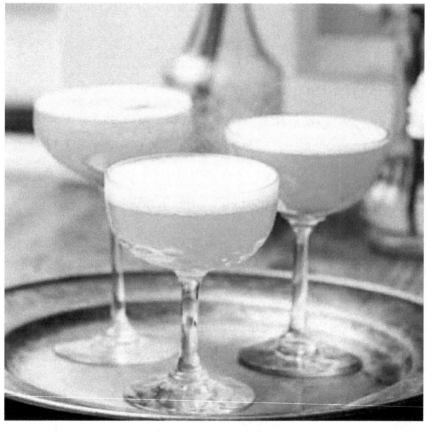

Makes: 8 Servings Prep Time: 10 minutes Cook Time: 15 minutes
Total Time: 25 minutes

INGREDIENTS:

1¾ cups (263 g) rhubarb,

Trimmed step and chopped

¾ cup (149 g) superfine sugar

Grated zest and juice of 1 orange

Chilled sparkling wine, to top off

PREPARATION:

Make rhubarb syrup. For this add sugar, orange zest, and rhubarb in a saucepan and add a splash of water. Bring it to the boil and simmer until rhubarb is soft.

Strain this mixture and get all the desired juice of rhubarb. Let it cool. Put a little amount of rhubarb syrup and pour wine over it.

NUTRITION

Calories: 125kcal | Carbohydrates: 22g | Protein: 1g | Fat: 1g | Sugar: 20g

# 50 Vegan Recipes

## ROASTED PUMPKIN QUINOA SALAD

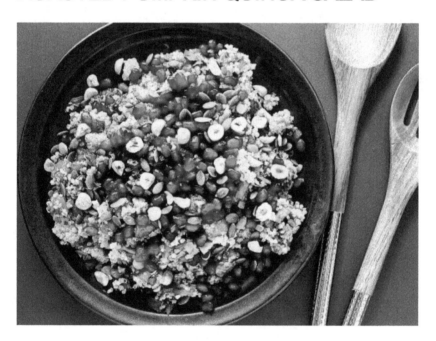

Total Time (prep time + cook time): 45 <u>minutes</u>

INGREDIENTS:

- Required for Roasted Pumpkin:

4 cups of cubed kabocha squash; buy at least a 1 ½-pound (680 g) squash

1 cup roughly chopped green parts of scallions

2 tablespoons of extra-virgin olive oil

1 tablespoon of maple syrup

1 teaspoon of ground coriander

1 teaspoon of well-grounded fennel seeds

½ teaspoon ground cumin

Kosher salt

Freshly ground black pepper

Quinoa & Salad:

¾ cup (68 g) washed quinoa, black, red, or white (we used white)

1 ½ cup (360 ml) water

¼ cup (8 g) finely chopped cilantro leaves

¼ cup (10 g) finely chopped mint leaves

2 tablespoons freshly squeezed lemon juice

1 tablespoon extra-virgin olive oil

1 teaspoon ground sumac

Kosher salt

Freshly ground black pepper

½ cup (90 g) pomegranate seeds

2 tablespoons raw or roasted pepitas

2 tablespoons roughly chopped peeled hazelnuts


PREPARATION:

For the Roasted Pumpkin:

Place a rack in the center of the oven. Preheat your oven to 425°F (220°C). Besides, align your half-sheet pan with aluminum foil and set aside.

Mix the pumpkin, scallions, oil, maple syrup, coriander, fennel, and cumin in a bowl so that all ingredients toss together well. Now add salt and pepper and scatter it in the pan in one layer.

Roast for 15 minutes and check then stir all ingredients and roast again for 10 to 15 minutes or until pumpkin is cooked. When it is done then set aside to cool and prepare the rest of the dish

For the Salad:

While the pumpkin is roasting, you can make the quinoa. Put water and quinoa in a small pot and add a pinch of salt. Now cover it and bring it to the boil. Cook until the water is absorbed. It takes around 10 minutes. When it is done turn off the heat but do not remove the cover. Allow to sit for 5 minutes, then fluff with a fork. Keep it at the side to cool down while you can make the rest of the dish.

Combine the cool pumpkin and quinoa in a bowl. Add olive oil, chopped herbs, lemon juice, and sumac. Now fold all ingredients gently so that all well-mixed together. Check the seasonings and add salt or pepper according to need. Set salad on a serving plate. Garnish the top with pomegranate, pepitas, and hazelnuts and serve.

NUTRITION

Calories: 230kcal | Carbohydrates: 28g | Protein: 5g | Fat: 12g |
Saturated Fat: 1g | Sodium: 4mg | Potassium: 31mg | Fiber: 4g |
Sugar: 5g | Vitamin C: 1mg | Calcium: 12mg | Iron: 1mg

# LOADED LOW FODMAP KALE CHIPS

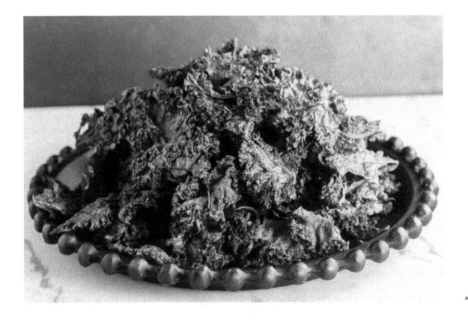

Prep Time: 10 minutes
Cook Time: 25 minutes

Total Time: 35 minutes

INGREDIENTS:

8- ounces (225 g) fresh curly kale, washed and dried

1 tablespoon olive oil, or Garlic-Infused Oil, made with olive oil

3 tablespoons nutritional yeast

1 teaspoon FreeFod Garlic Replacer

1 teaspoon smoked paprika

½ teaspoon FreeFod Onion Replacer

¼ teaspoon fine-grained table salt

1/8 teaspoon cayenne

1/8 teaspoon ground chipotle

PREPARATION:

Place two racks in your oven. Set both racks in the upper and lower third of the oven respectively. After this preheat your oven to 275°F (135°C). Besides, line parchment paper in two half-sheet pans and set aside.

First of all, you need to cut larger parts of the kale stems with a sharp paring knife. Now cut the kale into large pieces of around 2 to 3 inches. Put all pieces in a large mixing bowl.

Add oil over the kale and toss them with your other hand side by side. Drizzle oil on the leaves also so that all get evenly tossed.

Now it's time to coat the kale with all dry ingredients. For this, you need to mix all dry ingredients in a separate bowl. Add those dry ingredients over kale slowly and gradually. Mix and rub with your hands so that all kales can evenly coat with all ingredients. After this, set kale in a prepared pan as one layer.

Bake these kales for 10 minutes and then turn the pieces. Then, again bake for 10 minutes from another side of kales so that they can cook properly. Some of the edges might turn light brown, which is okay. Cool it down and serve.

NUTRITION

Calories: 87kcal | Carbohydrates: 25g | Protein: 6g | Fat: 4g | Saturated Fat: 1g | Sodium: 1mg | Potassium: 11mg | Fiber: 5g | Sugar: 1g | Vitamin A: 291IU | Iron: 1mg

# VEGAN LOW FODMAP KALE PESTO

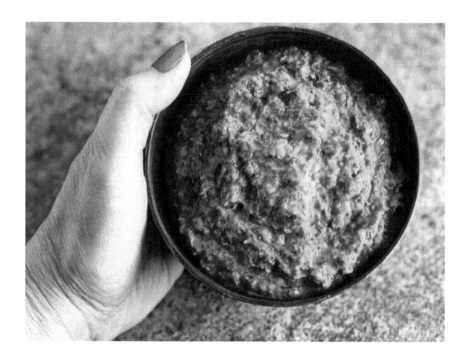

Prep Time: 5 minutes

Total Time: 5 minutes

INGREDIENTS:

Ounces (55 g) trimmed curly or Lacinato kale leaves; about 2 ½ cups chopped and lightly packed

½- ounce (40 g) basil leaves; about 1 cup lightly packed

½- ounce (40 g) flat-leaf parsley leaves; about 1 cup lightly packed

¼ cup (36 g) nutritional yeast, such as Bragg's

3 tablespoons lightly toasted pine nuts, see Tips

2 tablespoons freshly squeezed lemon juice

2 teaspoons FreeFod Garlic Replacer

½ teaspoon kosher salt

¼ cup (60 ml) extra-virgin olive

PREPARATION:

Add basil, kale, nutritional yeast, parsley, pine nuts, FreeFor garlic replacer, salt, and lemon juice in the food processor that is fitted with a metallic blade. Mince the greens finely by turning on and off the pulse. Add olive oil when the machine is in the process so that a smooth paste can be formed. Now, pesto is ready to use and you can refrigerate it for 1 week or can freeze it for 1 month

NUTRITION

Calories: 105kcal | Carbohydrates: 5g | Protein: 3g | Fat: 9g | Saturated Fat: 1g | Sodium: 146mg | Potassium: 10mg | Fiber: 1g | Sugar: 1g | Vitamin A: 149IU | Vitamin C: 2mg | Calcium: 2mg | Iron: 1mg

# ROASTED LOW FODMAP RATATOUILLE

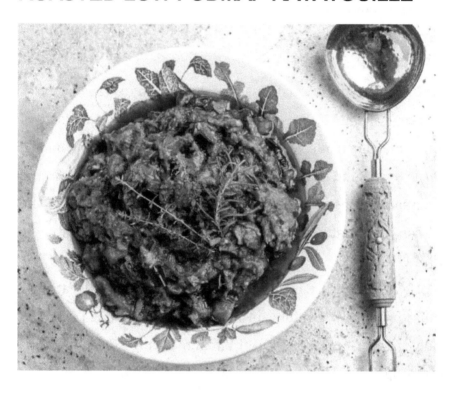

Prep Time: 20 minutes

Cook Time: 1 hour 30 minutes

Total Time: 1 hour 50 minutes

INGREDIENTS:

1 cup (64 g) roughly chopped scallions, green parts only

3 medium zucchini, about 8-ounces/225 g each, trimmed and cut crosswise into ¼-inch (6 mm) thick discs

2 medium eggplant, about 1-pound/455 g each, trimmed and cut into 1-inch (2.5 cm) cubes

3 red bell peppers, cored and cut into ¼-inch (6 mm) strips

Scant ½ cup (120 ml) Low FODMAP Garlic-Infused Oil, made with olive oil or purchased equivalent, plus more as needed

Kosher salt

3 small sprigs of fresh rosemary, plus extra as needed (see Tips)

6 fresh sprigs thyme, plus extra as needed (see Tips)

Kosher salt

3 large beefsteak tomatoes

1 teaspoon FreeFod Garlic Replacer

1 bay leaf

Freshly ground black pepper


PREPARATION:

Place three racks in your even with even distance. Then, preheat your oven to 350°F (180°C). Prepare three half-sheet pans for use. Spread the scallion greens and zucchini in one pan. Sprinkle oil and add salt according to taste. Make sure that oil is well coated on vegetables so that they do not burn. Place one small piece of rosemary along with 2 small springs of thyme on the top.

Spread eggplant on another pan in an even layer. Add oil and salt according to taste. Toss well to combine. Place one small piece of rosemary along with 2 sprigs of thyme on the top.

Spread the pepper strips on the third pan. Sprinkle oil and add salt according to taste. Mix well to combine. Place 1 small spring of rosemary and 2 small springs of thyme on the top.

Place all three pans in the oven and bake them for 45 minutes. While baking check vegetables once or twice and flip them on their pans. Roast until vegetables are cooked and beginning to shrink and have flavor inside them. Remove fresh herb stems when you take out the pans from the oven.

On the other side, bring a strainer over a large Dutch oven. Put a small pot on the stove and add water and bring it to a boil. Add tomatoes and cook for 1 minute or until the skin gets peel off. Remove and place it on the strainer. Cool it and remove the skin. Remove seeds and collect the juice in a Dutch oven. Add tomato flesh to the pot and squeeze it with your hands and discard the seeds.

Stir in the FreeFod Garlic Replacer. Now add all cooked vegetables in a Dutch oven. Add bay leaf and stir well by adding oil in it. Taste and add salt and pepper seasoning. Cook for about 30 minutes of low heat.

At this stage, everything is well-blend and well-mixed. At this point, the ratatouille is done. It is ready to eat but it is more tasteful on the 2nd or 3rd day.

NUTRITION

Calories: 191kcal | Carbohydrates: 14g | Protein: 3g | Fat: 15g | Sodium: 1mg | Fiber: 7g | Sugar: 6g

# NO FODMAP SAUTÉED CARROTS

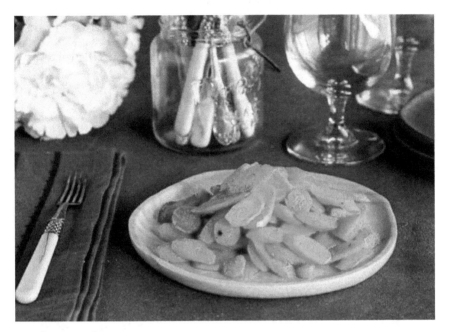

Prep Time: 5 minutes

Cook Time: 8 minutes

Total Time: 13 minutes

INGREDIENTS:

Pound (455g) trimmed orange carrots

2 tablespoons olive oil or Garlic-Infused Oil; optional

Kosher salt

Freshly ground black pepper


PREPARATION:

Peel the carrots and slice into ¼-inch ovals or rounds depending on your choice.

Place a pan on the stove and heat it well on low-medium heat. Add oil and coat all sides of the pan with oil. Now, add carrots and toss them well in oil. Saute these carrots for 3 to 5 minutes or until they are soft and crisp. Add salt and pepper according to taste and it is ready to serve.

NUTRITION

Calories: 123kcal | Carbohydrates: 13g | Protein: 2g | Fat: 7g | Fiber: 4g | Sugar: 7g

# NO FODMAP STEAMED POTATOES

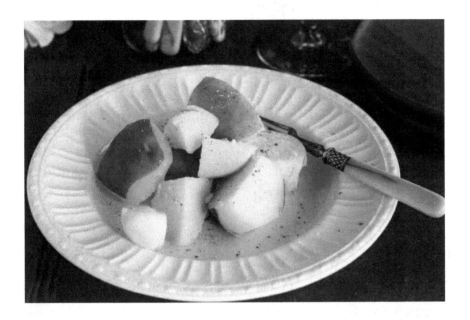

Prep Time: 10 minutes

Cook Time: 15 minutes

Total Time: 25 minutes

INGREDIENTS:

1 ½- pounds (680 g) potatoes such as red, white, yellow, or purple-skinned potatoes

Water

Olive Oil or Garlic-Infused Oil; optional

Kosher salt

Freshly ground black pepper

PREPARATION:

Wash the potatoes to make them clean. You can partially peel the skin or peel them completely. Cut the potatoes into bite-size cubes.

Fill a large pot with 1-inch water and place a steamer inside the pot. Position all potatoes in the steamer basket and cover it. Bring water to a boil. Cook for 10 to 15 minutes until potatoes get tender.

Take out potatoes and put them in a large bowl. Add salt and pepper according to taste. You can add little oil of your choice. It is done to serve.

NUTRITION

Calories: 131kcal | Carbohydrates: 30g | Protein: 3g | Fat: 1g | Saturated Fat: 1g | Sodium: 10mg | Potassium: 716mg | Fiber: 4g | Sugar: 1g | Vitamin C: 34mg | Calcium: 20mg | Iron: 1mg

# LOW FODMAP CHOCOLATE SORBET

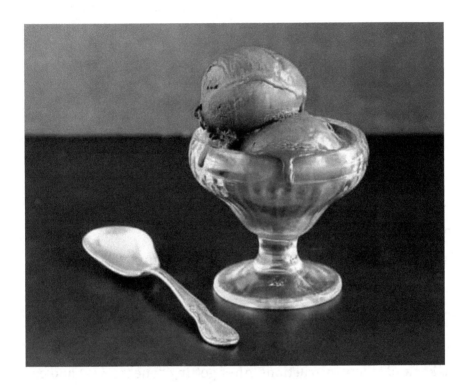

Prep Time: 5 minutes

Cook Time: 5 minutes

Chilling Time: 1 hour

Total Time: 1 hour 10 minutes

INGREDIENTS:

2 ½ cups (600 ml) water

1 cup (198 g) sugar

¾ cup (65 g) sifted Dutch-processed cocoa; Valrhona highly recommended

6- ounces (170 g) bittersweet or semisweet chocolate, very finely chopped; at least 60% cacao mass recommended

1 teaspoon vanilla extract

PREPARATION:

Add sugar, water, chocolate, and cocoa in a medium-sized saucepan. Mix ingredients together.

Boil this mixture on medium heat and then turn heat low. Simmer this mixture for 1 minute and whisk few times.

Turn off the heat and remove the pan. Strain it through a fine strainer. Whisk it with vanilla. Cool it at room temperature by stirring now and then. Put this mixture in a container and refrigerate it for 6 hours or overnight. Put it into the ice cream maker and follow instructions. After getting done freeze it and eat it in between 4 days.

NUTRITION

Calories: 234kcal | Carbohydrates: 47g | Protein: 2g | Fat: 6g | Sodium: 4mg | Fiber: 1g | Sugar: 39g | Calcium: 2mg

# LOW FODMAP STRAWBERRY GRANITA

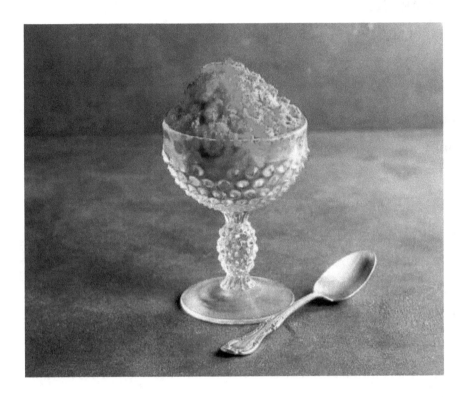

Prep Time: 20 minutes

Chilling Time: 1 hour 45 minutes

Total Time: 2 hours 5 minutes

INGREDIENTS:

Pounds (910 g) fresh strawberries, hulled and halved (or quartered if large)

1/3 cup (65 g) sugar

1 cup (240 ml) water

½ teaspoon lemon juice

PREPARATION:

First of all, you need to make a flat place in your freezer where a pan of 13 inches by 9 inches can be placed easily. Ready a pan to use.

Combine and stir strawberries and sugar together in a bowl. Mix until both get well-mixed and sugar is dissolved. It takes around 30 minutes.

Take out the juice of berries. Add water and lemon juice to it. Blend all ingredients and pass through the strainer and discard all the seeds.

Pour the strained strawberry mixture into your pan.

Freeze it until edges start to freeze. Use a fork and scorch frozen parts. Check again and again and get fluffy and icy crystals. Check every 30 minutes. Now it is ready to use or you can freeze and take out crystals before serving.

NUTRITION

Calories: 94kcal | Carbohydrates: 23g | Protein: 1g | Fat: 1g | Sodium: 2mg | Sugar: 18g | Vitamin C: 1mg

# LOW FODMAP ICED WHITE TEA WITH MANGO

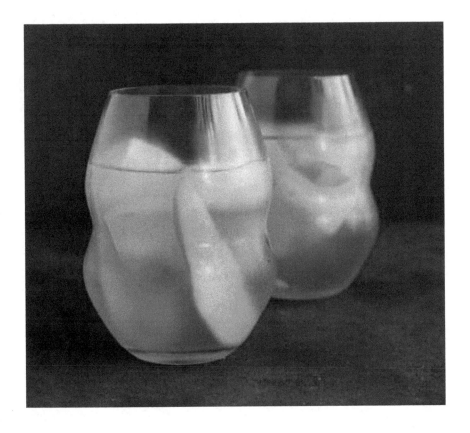

Prep Time: 5 minutes

Total Time: 5 minutes

INGREDIENTS:

Ice cubes

4 cups (960 ml) chilled brewed white tea

5 ¾- ounces (160 g) ripe mango flesh, cut into cubes or spear shapes

Simple Syrup, to taste

PREPARATION:

Add tea and ice cubes in glasses in an even amount. Add an even amount of mangoes and sugar according to taste. Stir it well and it is ready to serve.

NUTRITION

Calories: 28kcal | Carbohydrates: 7g | Protein: 1g | Fat: 1g

# LOW FODMAP CUMIN ALLSPICE DRY RUB

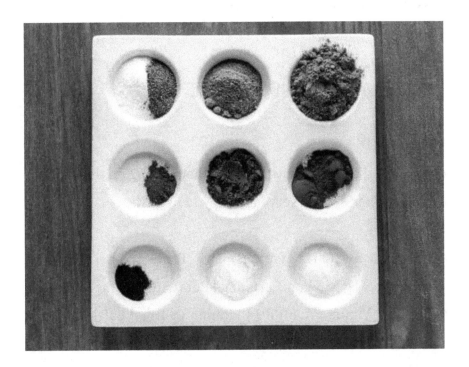

Prep Time: 5 minutes

Total Time: 5 minutes

INGREDIENTS:

¼ cup 24 g ground cumin

2 tablespoons ground coriander

2 tablespoons kosher salt

1 ½ teaspoon ground allspice

1 ½ teaspoon freshly ground black pepper

1 ½ teaspoons paprika

1 ½ teaspoon smoked paprika

1 teaspoon FreeFod Garlic Replacer

1 teaspoon FreeFod Onion Replacer

½ teaspoon cayenne

½ teaspoon ground chipotle

PREPARATION:

Add all ingredients to a bowl and mix them well. Add this mixture into a container and preserve it until you need it.

NUTRITION

Calories: 5kcal | Carbohydrates: 1g | Protein: 1g | Fat: 1g | Saturated Fat: 1g | Sodium: 1165mg | Potassium: 22mg | Fiber: 1g | Sugar: 1g | Vitamin A: 306IU | Vitamin C: 1mg | Calcium: 8mg | Iron: 1mg

# LOW FODMAP STRAWBERRY PEACH COCONUT CRISP

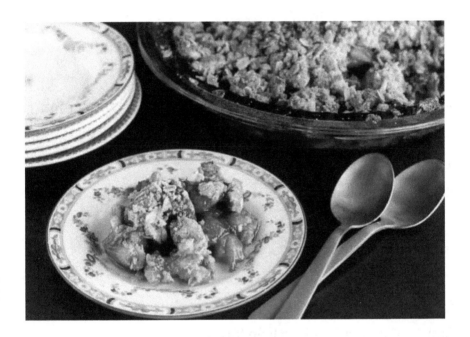

Prep Time: 10 minutes

Cook Time: 35 minutes

Total Time: 45 minutes

INGREDIENTS:

Fruit Filling:

Pounds (910 g) strawberries,

240 g chopped peaches, skin intact, stones discarded; buy 3 peaches to be safe

2 tablespoons cornstarch

2 tablespoons sugar

Crisp Topping:

1 batch Vegan Low FODMAP Crisp Topping, prepared and ready to use

½ cup (20 g) broad unsweetened coconut flakes

PREPARATION:

Place a rack in the mid of the oven and heat it to 375°F (190°C). Coat the inside of a ceramic pie dish with a non-stick spray and set aside.

For the Fruit Filling: Combine all strawberries and peaches in a large bowl. Add sugar and cornstarch and toss them well. Set aside and make the topping.

For the Crisp Topping: Toss the coconut chips into the prepared topping. Use your hands to help form nice clumps.

Assembly:

Spread prepared fruit mixture into prepared pan. Scatter the topping over the fruit and bake it for about 30 to 35 minutes. It is ready but let it sit for minutes before serving.

NUTRITION

Calories: 354kcal | Carbohydrates: 60g | Protein: 3g | Fat: 17g | Saturated Fat: 1g | Sodium: 1mg | Potassium: 173mg | Fiber: 3g | Sugar: 11g | Vitamin A: 14IU | Vitamin C: 67mg | Calcium: 18mg | Iron: 1mg

## LOW FODMAP PAPAYA LIME SORBET

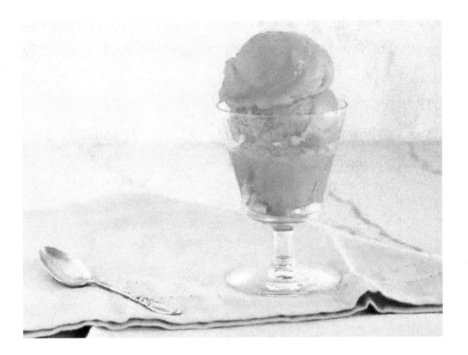

Prep Time: 10 minutes

Chilling Time: 7 hours

Total Time: 7 hours 10 minutes

INGREDIENTS:

Pounds (910 g) ripe papaya flesh,

Heaping ½ cup (99 g) sugar

¼ cup (60 ml) water

3 tablespoons freshly squeezed lime juice

PREPARATION:

Peel and cut papaya into a blender along with water, sugar, and lime juice. Blend this mixture well until smooth. After maxing, a mixture put it into a container and refrigerate it for 6 hours or overnight. Pour into ice cream maker and follow manufacturer's instructions. Freeze in an airtight container and eat preferably within 4 days.

NUTRITION

Calories: 42kcal | Carbohydrates: 11g | Protein: 1g | Sodium: 1mg | Fiber: 2g | Sugar: 7g

# LOW FODMAP BANANA COCONUT SORBET

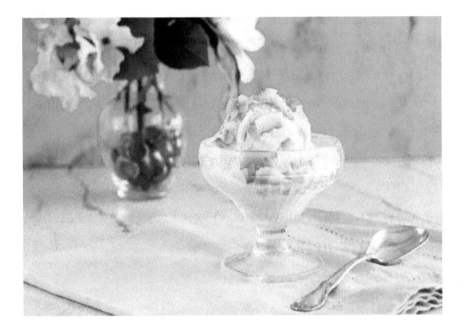

Prep Time: 10 minutes

Chilling Time: 7 hours

Total Time: 7 hours 10 minutes

INGREDIENTS:

13 to 14- ounce (370 g to 400 g) can of full-fat coconut milk

3 medium-sized, ripe bananas, peeled and cut into chunks

¼ cup (60 ml) light corn syrup, such as Karo, or to taste

1 tablespoon freshly squeezed lime juice, or to taste

½ teaspoon vanilla extract

Toasted Coconut Flakes; optional

PREPARATION:

Put the coconut milk, banana chunks, corn syrup, lime juice, and vanilla in a blender to blend them well. Blend all ingredients until smooth. Taste and add sweet or lime juice if you require more. Put it in an airtight jar and cool it.

Put it in the refrigerator for 6 hours or overnight. Take out and mix well before serving so that all ingredients are well-combined. Put it into an ice cream maker and follow the steps. Then, freeze it in the freezer and eat it in between 4 days.

NUTRITION

Calories: 97kcal | Carbohydrates: 13g | Protein: 1g | Fat: 5g | Sodium: 1mg | Fiber: 1g | Sugar: 6g

# LOW FODMAP PEACH ICED TEA

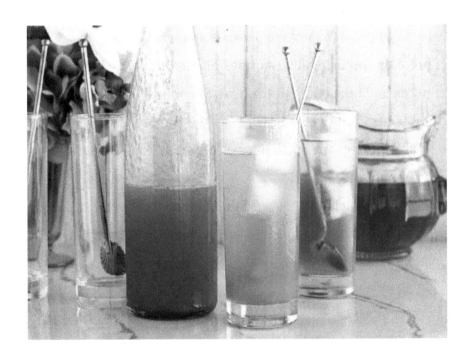

Prep Time: 15 minutes

Cook Time: 5 minutes

Steeping Time: 30 minutes

Total Time: 50 minutes

INGREDIENTS:

400 g chopped peaches, skin intact, stones discarded; buy 5 peaches to be safe

1 cup (240 ml) water

¾ cup (149 g) sugar

PREPARATION:

Wash your peaches and chop them. Discard all pits and get 400g flesh of your peaches. Mix the peaches along with sugar and water in a pot. Stir and bring it to simmer on medium heat. Simmer for 5 minutes and take off from the heat. Set it aside for 30 minutes. Put a fine strainer over a bowl. Pass the peach mixture through the strainer and get as much juice as possible. You can get around 2 cups of pure peach liquid.

Now to make peach iced tea, add the desired iced tea, and add ice in it. Also, add 2 tablespoons of pure peach juice and stir it well. It is ready to serve.

NUTRITION

Calories: 53kcal | Carbohydrates: 14g | Protein: 1g | Sodium: 1mg | Fiber: 1g | Sugar: 13g

# LOW FODMAP COLD BREW LATTE POPS

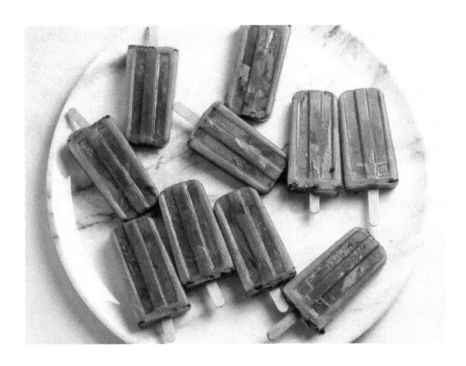

Prep Time: 10 minutes

Chilling Time: 8 hours

Total Time: 8 hours 10 minutes

INGREDIENTS:

2 1/3 cups (555 ml) cooled, strong brewed coffee

¾ cup (180 ml) full fat oat milk, such as Oatly

¼ cup (50 g) sugar; use superfine if you have it

3 tablespoons chocolate covered espresso beans, crushed, divided

PREPARATION:

Stir the coffee, oat milk, and sugar well together in a bowl. Whisk it until sugar dissolves.

Spread a small amount of the espresso beans at the bottom of your mold. Now fill your mold with the prepared coffee mixture and sprinkle leftover beans on the top. Now freeze it overnight and it is ready to serve.

NUTRITION

Calories: 48kcal | Carbohydrates: 9g | Protein: 1g | Fat: 1g | Sodium: 1mg | Sugar: 6g

# VEGAN LOW FODMAP CRISP TOPPING

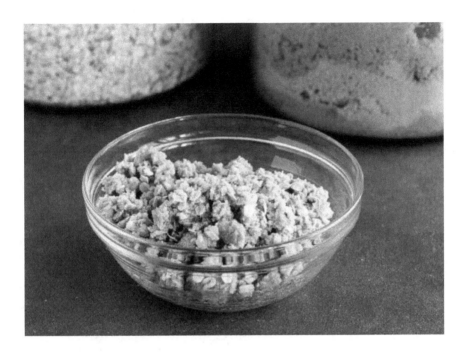

Prep Time: 10 minutes

Total Time: 10 minutes

INGREDIENTS:

¾ cup (160 g) firmly packed light brown sugar

¾ cup (109 g) low FODMAP gluten-free flour, such as Bob's Red Mill Gluten Free 1 to 1 Baking Flour

¾ cup (74 g) old-fashioned rolled oats (not instant or quick oats); use gluten-free if following a gluten-free diet

¼ teaspoon cinnamon

¼ teaspoon salt

½ cup (120 ml) melted coconut oil, either refined or unrefined

PREPARATION:

Add the brown sugar, flour, oats, cinnamon, and salt in a mixing bowl. Mix them well in a bowl by whisking. Now stir it in the melted oil so that all combine well. It is ready to freeze in a zip-top bag.

NUTRITION
Calories: 268kcal | Carbohydrates: 35g | Protein: 2g | Fat: 15g | Sodium: 73mg | Fiber: 1g | Sugar: 18g

# LOW FODMAP CHOCOLATE COCONUT SORBET

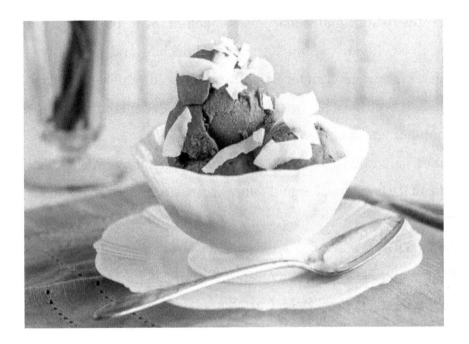

Prep Time: 15 minutes Cook Time: 5 minutes Chilling Time: 7 hours Total Time: 7 hours 20 minutes

INGREDIENTS:

1 cup (240 ml) water

¾ cup (149 g) sugar

6- ounces (170 g) finely chopped vegan semisweet or bittersweet chocolate; 60% cacao mass is perfect

1, 13 to 14- ounce (370 g to 400 g) can of full-fat coconut milk

½ teaspoon vanilla extract

Toasted Coconut Flakes; optional

PREPARATION:

Mix the water and sugar over medium heat until sugar is dissolved. Remove from heat, add chocolate and mix it well together. Now, let it sit for 5 minutes. Now add vanilla extract and whisk it well to make a smooth mixture. Put this mixture in a container and cool it.

Put this mixture in the refrigerator for 6 hours or overnight. Place it in an ice cream maker and follow instructions. Freeze it and eat it in 4 days.

NUTRITION

Calories: 262kcal | Carbohydrates: 36g | Protein: 1g | Fat: 13g | Sodium: 2mg | Fiber: 1g | Sugar: 32g

# LOW FODMAP PINEAPPLE WHISKEY BBQ SAUCE

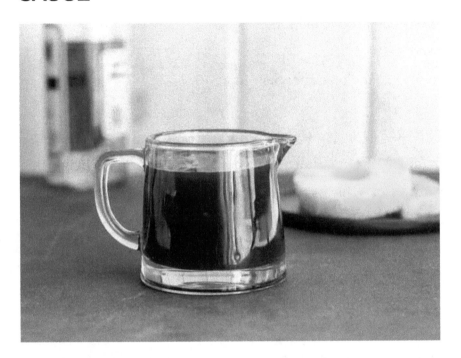

Prep Time: 5 minutes

Cook Time: 30 minutes

Total Time: 35 minutes

INGREDIENTS:

1 cup (240 ml) ketchup

1 cup (213 g) firmly packed light brown sugar

¾ cup (150 g) very finely chopped fresh pineapple, with any juices

¼ cup (60 ml) whiskey

3 tablespoons Unsulphured molasses

½ teaspoon FreeFod Garlic Replacer

½ teaspoon FreeFod Onion Replacer

½ teaspoon ground chipotle

Kosher salt

Freshly ground black pepper

PREPARATION:

Stir all of the ingredients together in a saucepan. Bring this mixture to a boil. Stir and simmer gently for 30 minutes until the mixture becomes thick and reduced. In the mid of stirring taste the sauce and add seasonings according to taste and start stirring again. The pineapple will have broken down almost to a sauce by the end of 30 minutes; no need to purée. It is ready to serve now.

NUTRITION

Calories: 61kcal | Carbohydrates: 14g | Protein: 1g | Fat: 1g | Saturated Fat: 1g | Sodium: 99mg | Potassium: 74mg | Fiber: 1g | Sugar: 13g | Vitamin A: 69IU | Vitamin C: 1mg | Calcium: 7mg | Iron: 1mg

# LOW FODMAP ICED BLACK TEA WITH LYCHEE

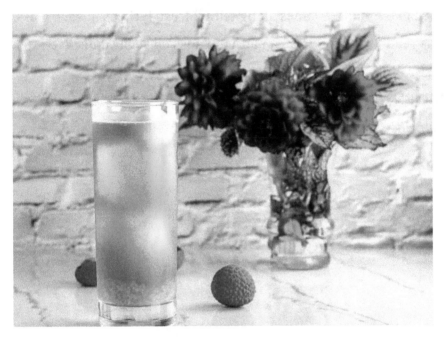

Prep Time: 5 minutes Total Time: 5 minutes

INGREDIENTS:

12 fresh lychees, peeled and pitted (120 g total)

Ice cubes

3 cups (720 ml) chilled brewed black tea

Simple Syrup, to taste

PREPARATION:

Take 8 fresh whole lychees and set aside. Take out the pure juice of remaining lychees through a blender or simply mash them with a fork.

Add chilled black tea in 4 separate glasses. Stir it in a pure into each glass. Add ice cubes along with 2 fresh lychees in each glass. It is ready to serve. You can add the desired sugar if needed after tasting it.

NUTRITION

Calories: 21kcal | Carbohydrates: 5g | Protein: 3g

# LOW FODMAP ICED GREEN TEA WITH PASSIONFRUIT

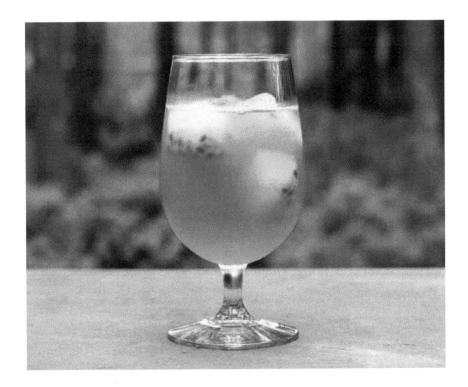

Prep Time: 5 minutes

Chilling Time: 8 hours

Total Time: 8 hours 5 minutes

### INGREDIENTS:

#### Passionfruit Ice Cubes:

- 2 ripe passionfruit

- 1 ice cube tray; ours has 16 wells

**Assembly:**

- 4 cups (960 ml) chilled brewed green tea

- **Simple Syrup,** TO TASTE

PREPARATION:

Cut passion fruit and take out the flesh with the help of a spoon. Put that flesh in the ice cube tray. Freeze it in a freezer until it is solid.

Add cubes in glasses. Pour chilled green tea in glasses equally. You can add more sugar syrup according to taste.

NUTRITION

Calories: 3kcal | Carbohydrates: 1g | Protein: 1g | Fat: 1g | Sodium: 1mg | Sugar: 1g

# LOW FODMAP BLACKBERRY PEACH CHUTNEY

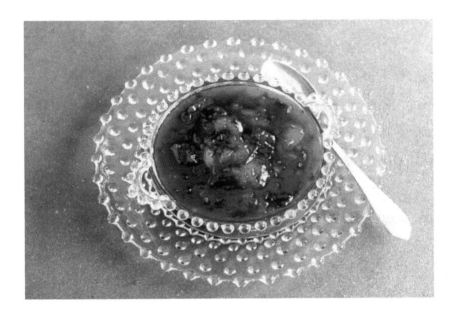

Prep Time: 10 minutes

Cook Time: 30 minutes

Total Time: 40 minutes

INGREDIENTS:

1 tablespoon vegetable oil

2 cups (128 g) chopped scallions, green parts only

240 g chopped peaches, peeled, stones discarded; buy 3 peaches to be safe

¾ cup (113 g) blackberries

¾ cup (160 g) firmly packed light brown sugar

1/3 cup (75 ml) apple cider vinegar

¼ teaspoon allspice

Kosher salt

Freshly ground black pepper

2 tablespoons lemon juice

PREPARATION:

Add oil to a pot and put it on medium flame. Add scallion greens and toss it in the oil for few minutes. Now add blackberries and peaches. Mash blackberries with the help of a potato masher. Saute for more few minutes on medium heat until fruit left the juice. Add allspice, sugar, and vinegar and stir well. Add also salt and pepper. Adjust heat and stir continuously until it gets thick. When it gets thick and completely mixed then remove from heat. Add lemon juice and stir it. Chutney is ready to serve immediately.

NUTRITION

Calories: 55kcal | Carbohydrates: 12g | Protein: 1g | Fat: 1g | Saturated Fat: 1g | Sodium: 1mg | Potassium: 17mg | Fiber: 1g | Sugar: 11g | Vitamin A: 16IU | Vitamin C: 2mg | Calcium: 2mg | Iron: 1mg

# LOW FODMAP GRILLED PINEAPPLE & KIWI SALSA

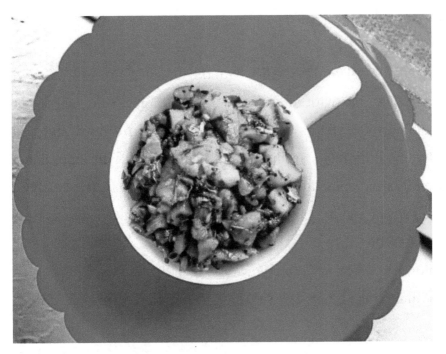

Prep Time: 10 minutes

Cook Time: 8 minutes

Total Time: 18 minutes

INGREDIENTS:

8- ounces (225 g) cored, pineapple rounds, about ½-inch (12 mm) thick

2 green kiwis, peeled and cut crosswise into ¼-inch (6 mm) discs

1 ½ tablespoon Onion-Infused Oil, made with vegetable oil or purchased equivalent

3 tablespoons finely chopped scallions, green parts only

2 tablespoons chopped cilantro

2 tablespoons lime juice

2 teaspoons minced jalapeno, or to taste

Kosher salt

PREPARATION:

Clean your grill and make fire with the help of charcoal. Toss kiwi and pineapples with oil and grill all vegetables. You need to get char marks on fruits. Cut and chop fruits in a bowl and add cilantro, lime juice, scallions, and jalapeno. Mix all ingredients well. Taste it and add seasonings according to taste. It is ready to use you can put it in a refrigerator.

NUTRITION

Calories: 37kcal | Carbohydrates: 6g | Protein: 1g | Fat: 2g | Sodium: 1mg | Fiber: 1g | Sugar: 1g | Vitamin C: 1mg

# LOW FODMAP PAPAYA SALSA

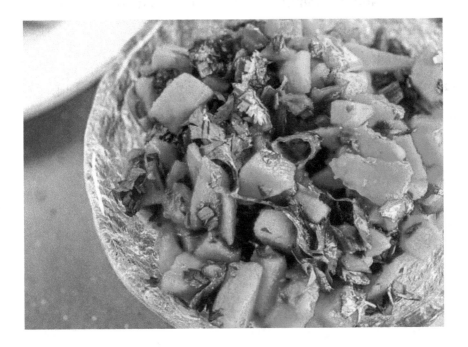

Prep Time: 10 minutes

Total Time: 10 minutes

INGREDIENTS:

12- ounces (340 g) ripe peeled papaya, diced

½ cup (16 g) chopped cilantro

½ cup (32 g) finely chopped scallions, green parts only

2 tablespoons lime juice

2 teaspoons minced jalapeno, or to taste

Kosher salt

PREPARATION:

Mix papaya, cilantro, scallions, lime juice, and jalapeno in a bowl. Toss all ingredients together until well combined. Taste and add seasonings as much required. Add more jalapeno if you like things hot. It is ready to use.

NUTRITION

Calories: 9kcal | Carbohydrates: 2g | Protein: 1g | Fat: 1g | Sodium: 1mg | Fiber: 1g | Sugar: 1g | Vitamin C: 1mg

# LOW FODMAP HUMMUS WRAP

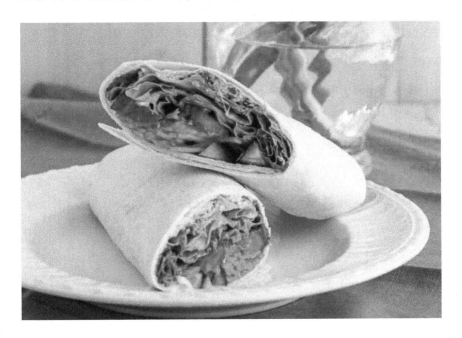

Makes: 1 Serving Prep Time: 10 minutes Total Time: 10 minutes

INGREDIENTS:

1, 10 to 12- inch (25 cm to 30.5 cm) low FODMAP gluten-free "flour-style" tortilla

2 tablespoons low FODMAP hummus

2 leaves butter lettuce

½ medium carrot, trimmed, peeled, julienned

½ Persian cucumber cut into thin sticks

½ beefsteak tomato, sliced into rounds

PREPARATION:

Take out your tortilla. Add and spread hummus all over the tortilla leaving a small corner at the top. Layer cucumber, carrot, and lettuce. Start rolling your tortilla from the bottom so that without hummus part comes at the top end. Squeeze the tortilla gently so that it can be rounded nicely. Wrap in plastic wrap and serve.

NUTRITION

Calories: 246kcal | Carbohydrates: 39g | Protein: 6g | Fat: 8g | Saturated Fat: 1g | Sodium: 2mg | Potassium: 71mg | Fiber: 3g | Sugar: 4g | Vitamin A: 994IU | Vitamin C: 1mg | Calcium: 11mg | Iron: 1mg

# VEGAN LOW FODMAP AVOCADO GREEN GODDESS DRESSING

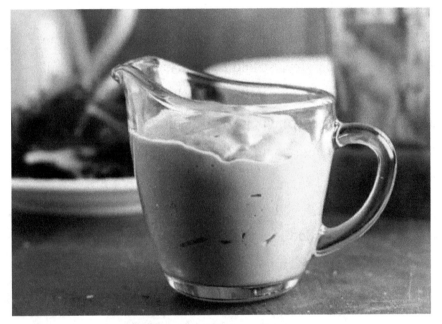

Makes: 5 Servings Prep Time: 5 minutes Total Time: 5 minutes

INGREDIENTS:

¼ cup to ½ cup (60 ml to 120 ml) warm water

2 tablespoons Garlic-Infused Oil, made with olive oil or purchased equivalent

1 tablespoon lime juice preferably fresh squeezed

Ounces (140 g) ripe avocado flesh, in chunks or pieces

¼ cup (8 g) parsley leaves

¼ cup (16 g) chopped scallions, green parts only

¼- ounce (7 g) fresh basil leaves

Kosher salt

Freshly ground black pepper

PREPARATION:

Add ¼ cup (60 ml) of warm water in a blender. Add oil, lime juice, avocado, parsley, scallions, and basil and blend all mixture well. Blend well until a smooth mixture is formed. Add seasonings of salt and pepper according to need. You can refrigerate it overnight in an airtight container.

NUTRITION

Calories: 93kcal | Carbohydrates: 3g | Protein: 1g | Fat: 9g | Saturated Fat: 1g | Sodium: 7mg | Potassium: 66mg | Fiber: 1g | Sugar: 1g | Vitamin A: 1071IU | Vitamin C: 17mg | Calcium: 19mg | Iron: 1mg

# VEGAN LOW FODMAP AVOCADO GREEN GODDESS VEGGIE SANDWICH

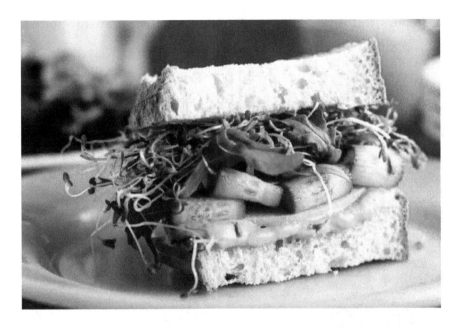

Makes: 1 Serving Prep Time: 5 minutes Total Time: 5 minutes

INGREDIENTS:

2 slices LOFO bread of choice

¼ cup (60 ml) Vegan Low FODMAP Avocado Green Goddess Dressing

¾ cup (30 g) alfalfa sprouts

Several leaves of fresh baby arugula

1 Persian cucumber, ends trimmed, cut into broad ribbons (I use a cheese planer or vegetable peeler)

1 slice vegan cheddar cheese, optional

PREPARATION:

Spread the Vegan Low FODMAP Avocado Green Goddess Dressing on the bread slices. Add a layer of cheese. Then add cucumbers, sprouts, and arugula. The sandwich is ready to serve.

NUTRITION

Calories: 338kcal | Carbohydrates: 41g | Protein: 9g | Fat: 15g | Fiber: 3g | Sugar: 4g

# NUTRITION FODMAP CHICKPEA SALAD

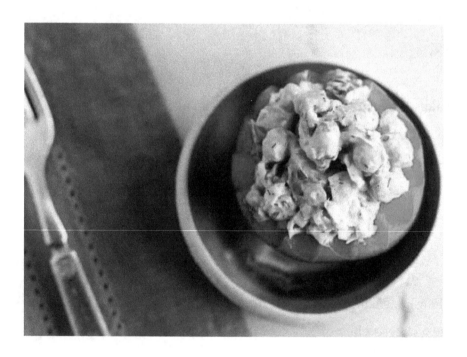

Makes: 8 Servings Prep Time: 10 minutes Total Time: 10 minutes

INGREDIENTS:

1, 15.5- ounce (439 g) chickpeas, drained, rinsed, and drained

1 medium carrot, trimmed and chopped into small dice

1 Persian cucumber, trimmed and chopped into small dice

¼ cup (16 g) finely chopped scallions, green parts only

2 tablespoons finely chopped flat-leaf parsley; optional

¼ cup (56 g) vegan mayonnaise

1 teaspoon Dijon mustard

1 teaspoon lemon juice

¼ teaspoon dried dill

Kosher salt

Freshly ground black pepper

PREPARATION:

Add chickpeas to a bowl and mash them with a fork. Add cucumber, carrot, and scallions. Mix all these along with mayonnaise, mustard, dill, and lemon juice. Add salt and pepper. The salad is ready to serve.

NUTRITION

Calories: 122kcal | Carbohydrates: 15g | Protein: 3g | Fat: 6g | Saturated Fat: 1g | Sodium: 49mg | Fiber: 1g | Sugar: 1g | Vitamin C: 1mg

# LOW FODMAP COLD SOBA SALAD WITH GREENS

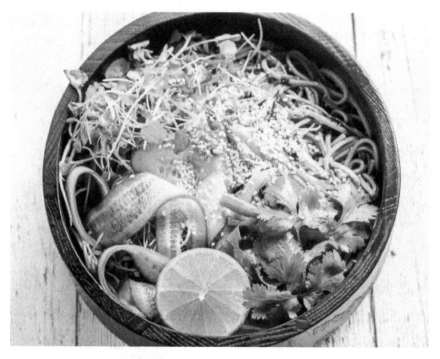

Makes: 4 Servings Prep Time: 10 minutes Cook Time: 8 minutes Total Time: 18 minutes

INGREDIENTS:

Ounces (115 g) soba noodles

Kosher salt

2 tablespoons low-sodium gluten-free soy sauce

1 tablespoon toasted sesame oil

1 tablespoon rice vinegar

¼ teaspoon Sriracha

1 cup (160 g) watercress, divided

3 scallions, green parts only, cut into long strips, divided

1 Persian cucumber, ends trimmed, cucumber cut into long, thin ribbons

1/3 cup (10 g) cilantro leaves

1 tablespoon toasted white sesame seeds

2 limes, cut in half crosswise

PREPARATION:

Boil soba noodles in salted water until all cooked. Rinse with cold water and drain it.

Stir together the soy sauce, sesame oil, rice vinegar, and Sriracha in a non-reactive bowl. Toss in the soba. Fold it in half of the watercress, scallions, and cucumber to coat. Divide this mixture into 4 bowls. Garnish each bowl with remaining ingredients and serve immediately.

NUTRITION

Calories: 164kcal | Carbohydrates: 28g | Protein: 7g | Fat: 5g | Saturated Fat: 1g | Sodium: 265mg | Potassium: 369mg | Fiber: 1g | Sugar: 1g | Vitamin A: 3218IU | Vitamin C: 31mg | Calcium: 94mg | Iron: 1mg

# Vegan Alfredo Sauce

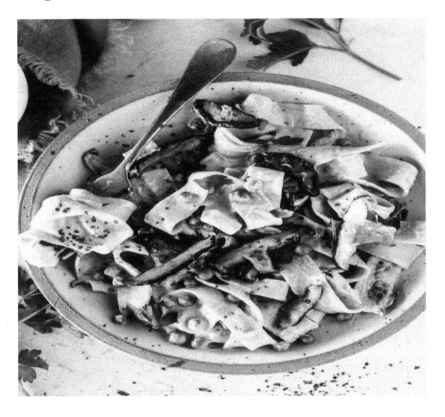

Time: 30 min

Ingredients

1–2 tablespoons olive oil

½ white onion

4 fat garlic cloves

½ cup raw cashews (or hemp seeds, see notes)

1 cup veggie broth (or 1 cup water and bouillon)

2 tablespoons nutritional yeast

½ teaspoon white miso paste

½ teaspoon salt

1/8 teaspoon nutmeg

5 ounces dry pasta, cooked to package directions

1 cup fresh peas (or frozen, or sub snow peas or steamed broccoli)

8 ounces mushrooms, sauteed, or try smoked mushrooms!

Garnish pepper, chili flakes, lemon zest ( Meyer lemons are especially nice), Italian parsley.

Instructions

Boil pasta in salted water. If using frozen peas then add them to the pasta water.

Make a sauce by heating oil over med-low heat. Add onion and garlic and saute them until tender and golden. Put them in a blender. Add cashews, veggie broth, nutritional yeast, miso, salt, nutmeg, and blend all ingredients until creamy and smooth.

Saute mushrooms in oil for 6 to 7 minutes. Toss them until they are golden brown.

Combine the cooked pasta along with sauce and gently warm it. Add mushrooms and mix well. Add in a bowl and garnish it.

Nutrition Facts

Amount Per Serving

Calories          564

Total Fat 21.2g          27%

Saturated Fat 3.5g

Cholesterol 0mg          0%

Sodium 676.7mg          29%

Total Carbohydrate 75.1g          27%

Dietary Fiber 9.2g          33%

Sugars 12.3g

Protein 23g          46

# Cucumber-Melon Soup

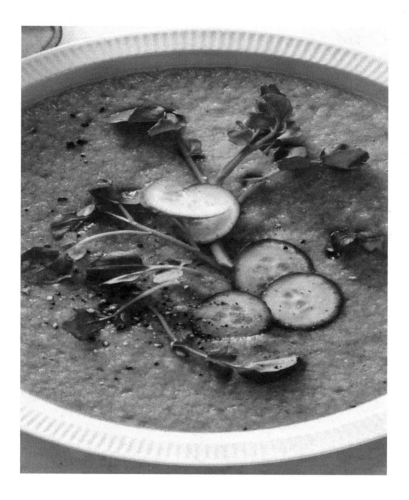

Time: 45 min

Ingredients

1 lb. English cucumbers, cut into pieces, plus more for serving

½ small honeydew melon, seeded and rind removed (about 1 pound), cut into pieces

½ c. flat-leaf parsley

3 tbsp. red wine vinegar

1 tbsp. fresh lime juice

2 tsp. sugar

Kosher salt and pepper

Watercress, for serving

Directions

In a blender add puree cucumbers, melon, parsley, vinegar, lime juice, sugar, and ½ teaspoon salt. Blend all these ingredients until a smooth paste is formed.

Put it in the refrigerator for about 1 hour. It is ready to serve.

Nutritional Information (per serving): About 75 calories, 0 g fat (0 g saturated), 3 g protein, 270 mg sodium, 18 g carbohydrate, 3 g fiber.

# Vegan Queso

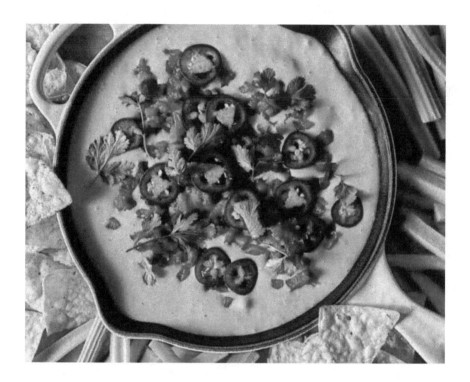

Time: 45 mins

Ingredients

2 large poblano peppers, halved and seeded

1 tbsp. olive oil

2 cloves garlic, pressed

1 c. cashews

2 tsp. chili powder

1 tsp. ground cumin

½ tsp. ground coriander

½ tsp. ground turmeric

Kosher salt and pepper

¼ c. nutritional yeast

Chopped cilantro and tortilla chips, for serving

Directions

Cut poblanos and boil them in a boiler. Boil them until they are charred. It takes about 3 to 5 minutes. Put them in a bowl and cover it. Remove the skin using a paper towel and cut peppers into bite-sized pieces.

On another side, heat oil and add garlic. Add spices and salt along with cashews. Add 1½ cups water and bring to a boil. Stir until cashews are tender.

After this add all mixture in a blender and add ½ cup water. Blend it well to form a smooth paste.

Add the blended mixture to a saucepan and cook until it gets thickened. Fold along with 2 poblanos. It is all set to serve with garnishing.

# Spinach, chickpea, and potato curry

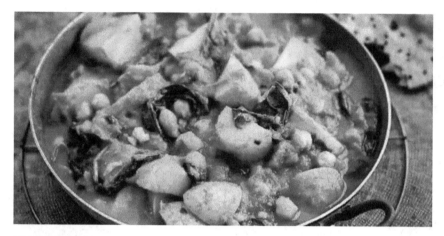

Time: 1 hour

Ingredients

Onion 1, chopped

Garlic 3 cloves, chopped

Ginger a thumb-sized piece, chopped

Green chili 1, chopped

Vegetable oil 1 tbsp

Ground cumin 1 tsp

Ground coriander 1 tsp

Ground turmeric 1 tsp

Chopped tomatoes 400g tin

Charlotte potatoes 400g, cut into chunks

Chickpeas 400g tin drained and rinsed

Spinach 100g, chopped

Lemon ½, juiced

Garam masala 1 tsp

Naans to serve

Method

Add garlic, ginger, onion, chili, and water in a blender. Blend it until a smooth paste.

Add oil and heat it. Add puree of onion and cook it until it gets reduced and brown. Now, add spices and cook it well. Add chopped tomato and cook again.

Add seasonings along with potatoes and chickpeas and water. Stir for about 30 minutes until potatoes are cooked. Add spinach and cook for some time.

Stir in the lemon juice and garam masala, and serve with naans.


Nutritional Information

Kcals 224

Fat 5.3g

Saturates 0.5g

Carbs 32g

Sugars 6.9g

Fibre 6.9g

Protein 8.8g

# Chili tofu ramen

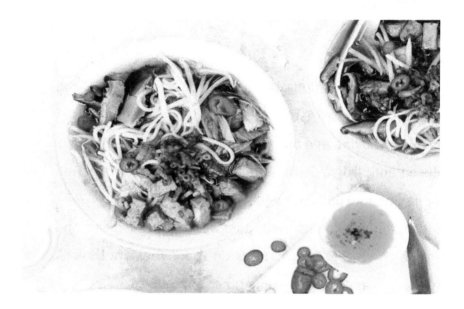

Time: 1 hour

Ingredients

Dried shiitake mushrooms 25g

Sake

Mirin

Soy sauce

Garlic 1 clove, bashed

Ginger thumb-sized piece, chopped

Red chilies 2, 1 sliced in half, 1 finely sliced

Winter greens (Pak Choy, kale, or spinach) 150g, shredded

Beansprouts 2 handfuls

Egg-free ramen noodles 300g

Marinated tofu 160g pack, cut into pieces

Chilli or garlic oil

Spring onions 2, finely sliced

Method

Add mushrooms, mirin and soy, the garlic and ginger, 1 tbsp each of sake, and the halved red chili in a large pan. Add 2 liters of water to it. Stir until the mushrooms get tender. Little mirin and soy sauce can be added to the season. Strain the stock into a clean pan and bring to a gentle simmer again. Cut the slices of mushrooms and remove the chili, ginger, and garlic. Blanch the greens and beansprouts and drain them well.

Heat the noodles in salted water. Cook until they get tender. Then, add it to 4 soup bowls.

Place the sliced mushrooms, greens, beansprouts, and marinated tofu in the stock for a few minutes. Add tofu and veg in the bowls, and pour over the stock. Add a few dots of chili oil, and scatter with spring onions and sliced chili, to serve.

Nutritional Information

Kcals 345

Fat 2.5g

Saturates 0.6g

Carbs 63.9g

Sugars 5g

Fibre 4.5g

Protein 13.6g

Salt 2.2g

## Orzo deli salad

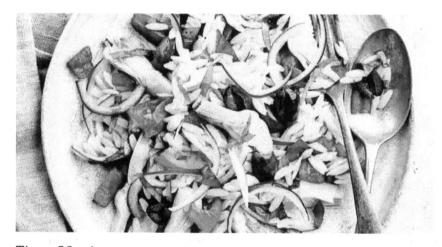

Time: 20 min

Ingredients

Red onion ½ small, finely sliced

Red wine vinegar 2 tbsp

Caster sugar a pinch

Orzo 100g (or other small pasta shapes)

Olive oil 2 tbsp

Roasted red peppers 2, chopped

Kalamata olives 12, halved and pitted

Artichoke hearts ½ small jar, drained and cut into wedges

SunBlush tomatoes 6, chopped

Basil a large handful, shredded

Method

Fold the onion with vinegar and sugar. Leave it aside and cook the pasta. Cook orzo by reading instructions and drain well.

Put olive oil and seasonings in the onion then tip in orzo and all vegetables. Add the basil and toss again.

Nutritional Information

Kcals 279

Fat 16.1g

Saturates 2.4g

Carbs 21.7g

Sugars 4.2g

Fibre 6.1g

Protein 8.8g

Salt 2.8g

# Courgetti som tam salad

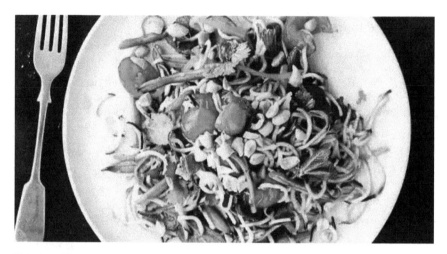

Time: 20 minutes

Ingredients

Courgettes 2

Carrot 1, shredded

Green beans 100g, cooked and cut into 8cm pieces

Cherry tomatoes 100g halved

Lime 1, juiced

Tamari 1, tbsp

Palm sugar or soft brown sugar 1 tbsp

Bird's eye chili 1, finely sliced

Coriander a small bunch, torn

Mint a small bunch, torn

Roasted peanuts chopped to make 1 tbsp

Method

Make long and thin courgette strands by using a spiraliser. Add these to a bowl with the carrot and green beans. Also put cherry tomatoes, lime juice, tamari, palm sugar, and chili in a mortar and mix with a pestle. Put this mixture on the courgette and marinate for 15 minutes.

Sprinkle the chop coriander and mint on the courgettes and mix well. It is ready to serve.

Nutritional Information

Kcals 177

Fat 5.1g

Saturates 0.9g

Carbs 20.3g

Sugars 17.7g

Fibre 7.5g

Protein 8.7g

Salt 1.7g

# Moroccan veg and chickpea tagine

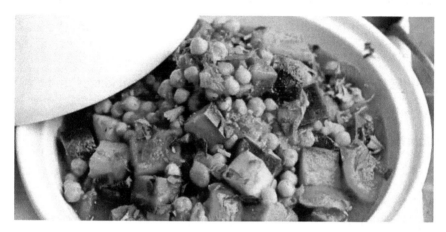

Time: 40 min

Ingredients

Red onion 1, chopped

Garlic 2 cloves, chopped

Spray olive oil

Ground cumin ½ tsp

Ground coriander ½ tsp

Ground cinnamon ½ tsp

Red pepper 1, seeded and chopped

Courgette 1, chopped

Aubergine 1, chopped

Vine tomatoes 4, chopped

Chickpeas 400g tin, rinsed and drained

Vegetable stock 250ml

Harissa 2 tbsp

Prunes 4, pitted and sliced

Flat-leaf parsley chopped to serve

Steamed couscous to serve (optional)

Method

Cut onion and put them in oil. Make them golden brown and add garlic. Now add all spices and toss well. Add all vegetables and cook until they change their color and you smell the fragrance of spices.

Put harissa, chickpeas, stock, and prunes and cook for 15 to 20 minutes. Add seasonings and cook until vegetables get tender. Sprinkle the parsley and it is ready to serve.

Nutritional Information

Kcals 187

Fat 3.6g

Saturates 0.5g

Carbs 24.6g

Sugars 14.1g

Fibre 11.7g

Protein 8.2g

Salt 0.3g

# Aubergine bhaji

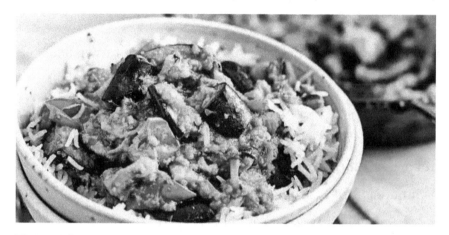

Time: 1 hour 10 min

## Ingredients

- **aubergines** 2, cut into chunks
- **groundnut oil**
- **onion** 1, roughly chopped
- **garlic** 2 cloves, roughly chopped
- **ginger** a walnut-sized chunk, peeled and chopped
- **cinnamon stick** 1/2
- **cardamon** 4 pods, squashed
- **cumin seeds** 2 tsp
- **green chilies** 2, chopped
- **ground turmeric** 1 tsp
- **ground coriander** 1 tbsp
- **ripe tomatoes** 4, chopped

- **tamarind paste** 2 tbsp

## Method

Heat aubergine in 2tbsp oil and 1tsp salt and toss well on medium heat. Cook until they are golden and soft. When the aubergine is tender then take it out.

Blend onion, garlic, and ginger in a blender. You can add a splash of water if needed.

Besides, add another tbsp of oil to the pan. When hot, add the cinnamon, cardamom pods, and cumin seeds and fry for a minute. Put the prepared onion paste and cook for about 5 minutes. Add all seasonings and cook for 2 more minutes. Cut tomatoes and add them to it. Cover with lid and cook for 10 minutes. Now, add the aubergine and simmer for another 10-15 minutes. It is ready to serve with rice.

Nutritional Information

Kcals 197

Fat 10g

Saturates 2g

Carbs 17.4g

Sugars 14.6g

Fibre 9.3g

Protein 4.6g

Salt 1.3g

## Smoked aubergine and pepper salad with pomegranate molasses

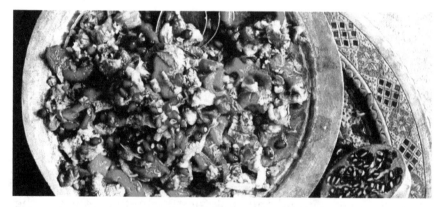

Time: 1 hour

Ingredients

Aubergine 4 large

Red pepper 3 large

Flat-leaf parsley a small bunch, roughly chopped (hold some back for the garnish

Garlic 2 cloves, crushed

Olive oil 6 tbsp

Lemon ½, juiced

Ground cinnamon a pinch

Pomegranate molasses 75ml

Pomegranate seeds 100g

Method

Remove the skins of aubergines and peppers either on the grill or on the hob. Heat them until they crisp and are completely charred. Under a hot grill, it will take 20 minutes. Once they are done set aside to cool them at room temperature.

Place the peppers into a plastic bag. Tie the bag for 20 minutes so that they get sweaty. The skin should be charred easily until you are left with flesh. Discard seeds and chop peppers and put them in a bowl.

Take out the flesh with the help of a metal spoon of aubergines and get the juice. Discard the charred skin. Chop into chunks and put them into a bowl.

Add all ingredients including parsley, crushed garlic, olive oil, lemon juice, cinnamon, salt, and pepper, and mix them well. It is ready to serve with garnishing.

Nutritional Information

Kcals 279

Fat 13.4g

Saturates 2.2g

Carbs 25.3g

Sugars 22.9g

Fibre 16.4g

Protein 6g

Salt 0.4g


## 39. coconut and peanut aubergine curry

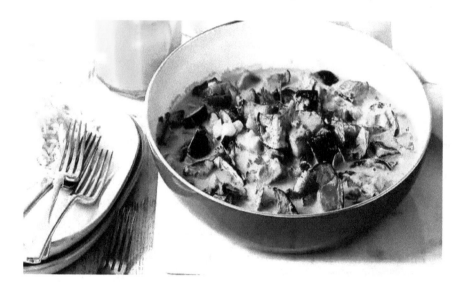

Time: 30 min

Ingredients

Oil for frying

Aubergines 2, cut into large chunks

Onions 2, chopped

Garlic 2 cloves, crushed

Ginger a 5cm piece, finely grated

Cumin seeds 1 tsp

Coriander seeds 1 tsp, crushed

Turmeric 1 tsp

Chilli powder ½ tsp

Half-fat coconut milk 400ml

Tamarind paste 1 tbsp

Peanut butter 1 tbsp

Coriander or bread or rice to serve

Method

Add 1 tbsp of oil to a pan and put aubergine. Cook then until they are golden and tender. Take them out once they are done

Cook onion in the same pan until they are golden and soft. Add the garlic and ginger and cook for a minute. Add the spices and cook for 2 minutes.

Now add peanut butter, coconut milk, and tamarind. Cook gently until peanut butter melts. Add the aubergine back and simmer for 15 minutes. Sprinkle coriander and serve it.

Nutritional Information

Kcals 251

Fat 15.5g

Saturates 7.2g

Carbs 17g

Fibre 10.6g

Protein 5.5g

Salt 0.1g

# Quick tamarind potato curry

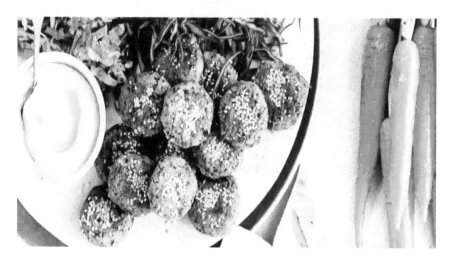

Time: 50 min

Ingredients

All-purpose potatoes like desirée or Elfe 750g, peeled and cut
into large dice

Onion 1, large

Garlic 1, clove

Ginger a walnut-sized chunk, roughly chopped

Green chili 1, chopped

Oil for frying

Cumin seeds 1 tsp

Fennel seeds ½ tsp

Ground coriander 1 tsp

Medium chili powder 1 tsp

Plum tomatoes 400g tin

Brown sugar 2 tsp

Tamarind paste 2 tbsp

Coriander a large handful

Rice or naan bread to serve

Method

Put potatoes in a pan and add salted water. Boil these potatoes and take them out. Blend garlic, ginger, onion, chili, and 2 tbsp of water to make a puree.

Add oil to a pan. Add onions and cook them until they are tender. Add all spices and cook. Add puree and cook for 5 minutes. Put tomatoes, tamarind, and sugar and cook for 10 minutes. Add boiled potatoes and a little water. Cook until potatoes are completely cooked. Serve with rice or naan.

Nutritional Information

Kcals 255

Fat 4.2g

Saturates 0.4g

Carbs 45.3g

Sugars 12.6g

Fibre 6.2g

Protein 5.7g

Salt 0.4g

# Carrot falafel

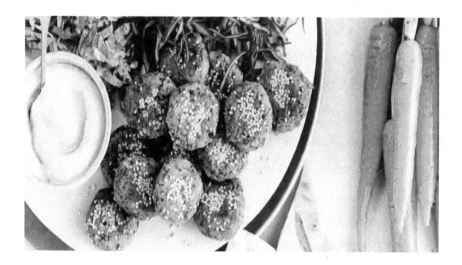

Time: 50 min

Ingredients

FALAFEL

Chickpeas 1 tin, drained and dried on kitchen paper

Carrots 100g, peeled and grated, excess moisture squeezed out

Garlic ½ clove, crushed

Ground cumin ½ tsp

Ground coriander ½ tsp

Coriander 1, handful, chopped

Cornflour 1 tbsp

Sesame seeds to coat

Oil for frying

TO SERVE

Finely shredded lettuce

Finely shredded red cabbage tossed in lemon juice

Whole pickled chilies

Tomato wedges

Hummus

Lemon wedges

Hot sauce

Middle Eastern flatbreads

Method

Add first 7 ingredients along with 1 tsp of sea salt into a blender and blend to make a smooth paste.

Form large tablespoons of the mix into flattish balls. Put on a lined baking sheet and chill for 30 minutes. Sprinkle with a few sesame seeds and pat into the surface to stick.

Put a small amount of oil in a pan and heat it. Fry falafels and cook them until they are crisp and golden.

Nutritional Information

Kcals 345

Fat 18.5g

Saturates 1.9g

Carbs 28.9g

Sugars 4g

Fibre 9.5g

Protein 10.8g

Salt 2.5g

---

# Vietnamese-style green soup

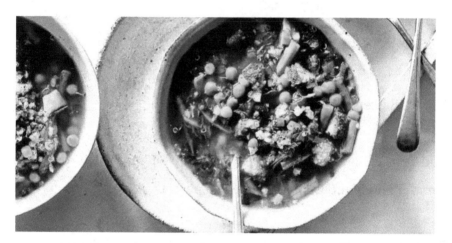

Time: 30 min

Ingredients

Olive oil 1 tbsp

Spring onions 1 bunch, chopped (including green bits)

Lemongrass 1 stalk, woody outer leaves removed, finely chopped

Ginger a walnut-sized chunk, finely chopped

Garlic 1 clove, crushed

Red chili 1, finely chopped

Quinoa 3 tbsp

Vegetable stock 1 liter

Broccoli 100g, chopped into 1cm pieces

Green beans 100g, chopped into 2cm pieces

Frozen peas 100g, defrosted

Spinach 100g, shredded

Basil a handful, chopped

Mint a handful, chopped

Lime 1, zested and juiced

Method

Add oil to a pan and heat it. Add lemongrass, ginger, chili, garlic, and spring onions. Cook them for 3 to 4 minutes. Add the quinoa and stock, and simmer until the quinoa is tender. Add the broccoli and beans, and cook for 3 minutes. Add the peas and spinach, and cook for another 2 minutes. Add seasonings and serve.

Nutritional Information

Kcals 134

Fat 4.5g

Saturates 0.6g

Carbs 14.1g

Sugars 5.9g

Fibre 5.9g

Protein 6.3g

Salt 0.6g

# Low FODMAP Cold Soba Soup with Watercress and Radishes

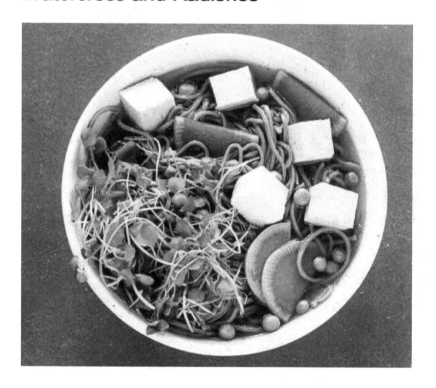

Makes: 4 Servings Prep Time: 10 minutes Cook Time: 10 minutes Total Time: 20 minutes

INGREDIENTS:

8- ounces (225 g) extra-firm tofu, drained

4- ounces (115 g) soba noodles

¼ cup (60 g) frozen, defrosted peas

3 cups (720 ml) Low FODMAP Vegetable Broth, chilled

3 tablespoons low-sodium gluten-free soy sauce

2 tablespoons rice vinegar

1 teaspoon toasted sesame oil

1 teaspoon sugar

½ teaspoon minced fresh ginger

2 cups (160 g) watercress

3- ounces (85 g) white daikon radish, peeled and thinly sliced crosswise, then cut crosswise

2 tablespoons minced scallions, green parts only

Sriracha

Cut tofu into pieces. Fold pieces in a paper towel and place any heavy object on top of tofu cubes. In this way, excessive water will be drained.

Meanwhile, boil noodles and peas in salted water. When done then drain and rinse through cold water.

Put noodles among bowls evenly. Whisk together the chilled broth, soy sauce, rice vinegar, sesame oil, sugar, and ginger until sugar is dissolved. Pour over noodles. Serve it by garnishing it with tofu.

NUTRITION

Calories: 205kcal | Carbohydrates: 31g | Protein: 14g | Fat: 4g | Saturated Fat: 1g | Sodium: 273mg | Potassium: 462mg | Fiber: 1g | Sugar: 2g | Vitamin A: 3775IU | Vitamin C: 51mg | Calcium: 152mg | Iron: 1mg

# Low FODMAP Peanut Lime Sauce

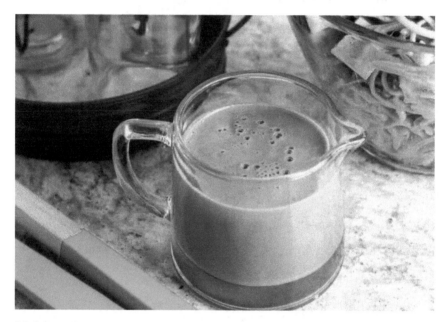

Makes: 8 Servings Prep Time: 5 minutes Total Time: 5 minutes

INGREDIENTS:

½ cup (120 ml) Garlic-Infused Oil, based on vegetable oil or purchased the equivalent

½ cup (120 ml) low sodium, gluten-free soy sauce

½ cup (120 ml) apple cider or rice vinegar

½ cup (134 g) smooth peanut butter, either natural or no-stir style

¼ cup (60 ml) freshly squeezed lime juice

¼ cup (60 ml) toasted sesame oil

2 scallions, green parts only, roughly chopped

2 tablespoons firmly packed light brown sugar

2 tablespoons minced fresh peeled ginger

Water, if needed

Preparation:

Add all of the ingredients to the blender. A lot of water is required to blend the peanut butter. Blend until the mixture turns into a smooth and soft paste. The sauce is then ready to serve.

NUTRITION

Calories: 300kcal | Carbohydrates: 10g | Protein: 5g | Fat: 29g | Fiber: 1g | Sugar: 5g

CPSIA information can be obtained
at www.ICGtesting.com
Printed in the USA
LVHW012345060621
689536LV00002B/109

9 781802 102505